# My Patients and Other Animals

# My Patients and Other Animals

## A Veterinarian's Stories of Love, Loss, and Hope

*Suzy Fincham-Gray*

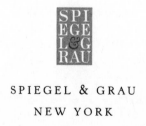

SPIEGEL & GRAU

NEW YORK

Published in the United States by Spiegel & Grau, an imprint of Random House, a division of Penguin Random House LLC, New York.

SPIEGEL & GRAU and colophon is a registered trademark of Penguin Random House LLC.

LIBRARY OF CONGRESS CATALOGING-IN-PUBLICATION DATA
Names: Fincham-Gray, Suzanne, author.
Title: My patients and other animals: a veterinarian's stories of love, loss, and hope / by Suzanne Fincham-Gray.
Description: New York: Spiegel & Grau, [2018]
Identifiers: LCCN 2017025329 | ISBN 9780812998184 (hardback) | ISBN 9780812998191 (ebook)
Subjects: LCSH: Fincham-Gray, Suzanne. | Veterinarians—Biography.
Classification: LCC SF613.F528 A3 2018 | DDC 636.089092 [B]—dc23
LC record available at https://lccn.loc.gov/2017025329

Printed in the United States of America on acid-free paper

randomhousebooks.com
spiegelandgrau.com

2  4  6  8  9  7  5  3

Book Design by Jo Anne Metsch

FOR ROB AND WREN

*I love you as high as the sky until it says stop.*

# Contents

# Author's Note

These stories are true, but memory is fallible. This memoir reflects the author's present recollections of past events. Some names and characteristics have been changed, some events have been compressed, and some dialogue has been re-created. Nevertheless, the author has always strived to represent the essential truth.

# My Patients and Other Animals

# Peter and the Horse

Trees lining the country lane forced the air into an irregular rhythm that buffeted my eardrum through the Land Rover's open window. Sunlight flitted through branches, splashing the windscreen with unpredictable brilliance. The clean, savory perfume of the cow parsley clustered in the passing hedgerow mingled with the less subtle notes of manure clinging to my clothes. Beneath my stocking feet lay my lunch, along with empty syringe casings, odd scraps of paper with medical notes, and less identifiable detritus from our day's farm calls in the Herefordshire countryside. And beside me, expertly guiding the SUV around the twists and turns of the narrow lane, sat Peter, the large-animal veterinarian with whom I was "seeing practice"—the UK term for gaining experience as a veterinary student by shadowing veterinarians in various settings.

We slowed, and Peter maneuvered the Land Rover into a gateway with a narrow dirt turnout that led to a long paddock running next to the road. There was one small gray pony in the field. We got out and walked to the back of the SUV, where I removed a pair of khaki Wellington boots and bottle-green coveralls from the boot. Peter was already suited up and pulling on his wellies with practiced ease by the time I'd unfolded my outfit. I stuffed the too-long pant legs into my socks before stepping into my wellies, holding on to the car for balance.

Shuffling around in the boot, he located a black case the size of a laptop beneath the piles of syringes, rectal examination gloves, medication bottles, and shiny stainless steel implements that made me want to cross my legs. Peter opened the case to reveal what looked like an old-fashioned pistol. Made from blackened metal, it was small and sturdy with a brown wooden handle. The grip had the patina of age, cured by the skin oils embedded in its crosshatch. It was the sort of thing I imagined from back in the Wild West, thousands of miles from this English field. Alongside the gun was a box of ammunition that served one specific purpose. This was a single-shot pistol, and I was about to shoot my first horse.

I had been volunteering at the small-animal clinic in the veterinary practice that Peter co-owned since I was fourteen, when my determination to become a vet had driven me to make weekly visits to observe Peter's small-animal partner, George, conducting his evening surgery.

The practice was a ten-minute walk from my childhood home in Hereford, a small cathedral city nestled on the Welsh border. In autumn, the short trek to the clinic was scented by delicious, yeasty apples fermenting at the cider factory across the street. During the spring, I was accompanied by the woolly odor and noise from trucks full of sheep and cattle on their way to market.

I'd logged hours upon hours in the small-animal clinic, watching vaccination after vaccination, cleaning hundreds of cages and walking every conceivable size of dog.

George was a Scotsman with a booming brogue and generous stature, both of which were barely contained by the thin walls of the consulting room. The clinic was in a converted Edwardian house, and the waiting area, which had presumably once been the drawing room, was always filled with eager owners and nervous pets awaiting their turn with the "Scottish vet." After each appointment, George would stand in the doorway, his shoulders filling the frame, and call out for his next client in the high-pitched, slightly girlish tone he used to talk to his patients. Every consultation started the same way: "Hello, Mrs. Jones. How are you and Fluffy doing this lovely evening?" And he would narrate the entire visit: "Just a wee poke," when administering a vaccine; "We'll be in and out in a flash," when describing a surgery. Medications were prescribed by color and shape rather than their pharmacology. His parting words to every owner were "Take them home and love them."

Over the years I'd heard all of George's jokes and grown impatient at the unscientific language he used with his clients—I aspired to learn the precise name and clinical description of every disease—but I'd bided my time in anticipation of the moment Peter would invite me into the passenger seat of his Land Rover. And, finally, after four years of formal veterinary education, I had graduated from my unobtrusive corner of the exam room to the passenger seat, ready to visit horses, cows, sheep, and any other beast too big or messy to fit into a consulting room. Now it was my turn to entertain high school volunteers in the kennel room with tales of calving successes, hoof trimming, and cesarean sections—the same stories I had once listened to with rapt, jealous attention.

Although my upbringing was essentially urban—if a city with a one-screen cinema, a handful of shops, a nightclub called Marilyn's, and a Pizza Hut was considered urban—the countryside Peter and I traveled through was familiar. It was where my family took walks through bluebell-carpeted woods in spring, picked strawberries in summer, and stomped through piles of crunchy autumn leaves. The gamboling lambs, grazing cattle, and hard, stiff earth of a plowed winter field had once been little more than fun distractions. But riding with Peter on large-animal calls, visiting farms for TB testing, calving, and managing herd healthcare, I had come to realize how integral farming was to my home.

Peter was well known in Herefordshire—with his muttonchops, and his cravat and collared shirt regardless of the day's duties. He was no match for George in physical stature, but he occupied an equally substantial place in the practice and community. Peter's energy was suited to the outdoors; his wiry forearms and strong grip were made for wrangling horses' hooves, not tending to soft kittens' paws. He carried the vaguely aloof brusqueness and rounded vowels of a country gentleman, and I felt naïve and weighed down by my need to prove myself in his presence. Over the prior two weeks of our working together we'd developed a good, if slightly distant, rapport. Compared to George and his jovial bedside manner, Peter had a more formal approach. But the rigor with which we discussed timely topics in veterinary medicine, and our meticulous daily reviews of clinical practice, more than made up for the lack of amiable banter.

We were visiting a pony who was no longer eating. Peter, who'd examined her before, suspected lymphosarcoma, a cancer of white blood cells. Her owners had declined further diagnostics and treatment—and to be present for this final visit. I didn't remember the pony's name. Peter had told me a few miles back, but it had instantly skidded from my mind. My thoughts were desperately clinging to the scientific and clinical aspects of the visit. I wanted to know her name, though, to gently whisper it under my breath once I stood in front of her. But more than that, I wanted to appear calm and composed. I couldn't bring myself to ask.

My childhood was littered with mostly imaginary animals. Despite my best attempts to convince my parents that a dog was an essential family member, I had to make do with stuffed toys and wheeled suitcases as companions. On one summer family vacation in a remote, soggy corner of Wales, I even adopted a pet rock, complete with a

collar and leash fashioned from long-abandoned red twine. Unfortunately, my parents did not share my enthusiasm for my new pet, and
I was forced to abandon her at the end of the trip, leaving only my
dad's endless apocryphal stories of his childhood puppy, Patch, to satisfy my dog-owning ambition.

Patch had been a black-and-white Border collie with a penchant
for getting into trouble, and tales of him chewing through electrical
cords, jumping out of a moving car's window, and dining on the contents of the compost heap were part of our family lore. Patch had
died of old age when my dad was a teenager, but even decades later,
it often seemed like he was about to trot into the room.

My dad was a dog person and, for as long as I could remember, I
had wanted to be like him, right down to wishing that his exuberant
caterpillar eyebrows would one day meet in the middle of my forehead. While my mum's teaching career held no mystery—I went to
school every day; I knew what teachers did—my dad was a microbi-
ologist in a veterinary laboratory. And, because he wasn't occupied
with keeping two girls fed, clothed, and clean along with holding
down a full-time job, he was the parent who taught me how to ride a
bike, tell a joke, look down a microscope, and what the offside rule in
football meant. He was also an eager amateur photographer, and for
a time our attic contained not only the precisely-to-scale model rail-
way he spent hours researching, painting, and setting up, but also the
red-lit mystery of a darkroom. Once I was old enough to be trusted
around the shallow trays of alchemical liquids, I would hover close to
my dad in the small space, enthralled, while pictures developed on
previously stark sheets of photographic paper.

Ultimately, it was a simple picture that my dad took of a laboratory sink, discolored with the residue of dyes he'd used to stain microscopic specimens, that illuminated my gateway into the world of
science. I remember the first exhilarating instant I saw the image, the
flat grayness of the once-white sink, the swirling blues, purples, and
pinks curling around the drain in confusing whorls. I was fascinated,

hooked. It was a visual representation of the days my dad spent culturing microscopic organisms on agar plates and in flasks of nutrient broth—the type of scientific life I wanted to be a part of.

When I was fourteen, my interest crystallized into a determination to join the world of veterinary medicine. The mystery of abdominal cavities revealed by a scalpel and the secrets of bones discovered on X-rays were calling to me. I was entranced by the science of physiology and disease—how bodies work, get broken, and are fixed again. I wasn't inspired by a family pet saved from the brink of death by a plucky veterinarian—my rock was indubitably resilient—and I couldn't tell heartening stories of baby birds I'd nursed back to life from certain doom. My motivation came down to a picture of a dirty sink and a wonder at what lay beyond the plug hole.

Despite my uncommon inspiration, my dream of becoming a veterinarian was not unusual. The bucolic, very English portrayal of veterinary medicine in *All Creatures Great and Small*, a 1980s BBC series based on James Herriot's books, inspired millions every Sunday evening to consider the same path. The show was set during the 1940s and '50s in a fictional North Yorkshire village. The countryside was rolling and unspoiled, and the heroes—James and the younger Tristan Farnon—dashing and brave. It was a halcyon place of small, neat stone cottages with meticulously planted gardens, and a pub where the gents drank pints of local ale while the ladies sipped tea at the vicarage.

Herriot's veterinarian was the center of a thriving agricultural community, driving from farm to farm delivering calves, treating lame horses, and performing the occasional house call for a rich landowner's over-pampered Pekingese. Women were wives and assistants, and veterinary medicine, in Herriot's time, was a male-dominated, large-animal-focused profession. It was, after all, only a few decades earlier, in 1922, that Aleen Cust, the first British female veterinarian, was finally permitted to practice, twenty-five years after she'd completed her studies.

The tide, however, was turning. And by the mid-1990s, when I began veterinary school, two-thirds of my classmates were female. Despite this shift, the majority of the veterinarians I met seeing practice, and the senior lecturers and clinicians at university, were male. When I went on farm calls with Peter, my presence and my introduction as a vet student were sometimes met with skepticism and outright sexism. Peter and George showed no such prejudice, but I desperately wanted to avoid giving anyone proof that I couldn't do a man's job, especially when it came to holding a gun against a horse's head and pulling the trigger.

When I started seeing practice with Peter—the summer before the final year of my veterinary education—I had not yet killed an animal. Although I'd stood a respectful distance from the cats and dogs I'd seen euthanized, passively witnessing their last breath, I had chosen not to look too closely at this aspect of my future career. I knew it was something I would do—would have to do—and I'd heard veterinarians talk about how it was *the best decision* for a suffering pet. But I'd never pictured myself administering the fatal bullet to a sick horse. I was so caught up in studying the factual, scientific nature of disease that I'd barely had time to consider the practical applications for my patients.

Four years of vet school separated the teenager who'd hovered in the corner of the examination room from the student who stood in that field. When I moved to London for my first year at university I'd just turned nineteen. I was staying in Commonwealth Hall, a large intercollegiate residence. My dad had driven me the three hours east from Hereford to London. As the view through the car window changed from the countryside of my childhood to the monotonous gray of the motorway, my excitement shifted into a tugging dread that made me want to beg him to turn the car around. Instead, I complained about his taste in music and argued with him about which cassette to put in the player.

After we'd decanted the contents of the boot and backseat into my cupboard of a room, I realized that the clod that had been slowly thickening in my throat all afternoon was going to make it difficult to say goodbye. A swift survey of my home for the next year had done little to raise my spirits—a single bed with institutional sheets and a thin, lumpy duvet; a radiator covered in multiple layers of peeling paint; a small wardrobe that smelled of other people's clothes; a faux wood desk with the edges chipped and cracked; and, wedged in the corner, a tiny sink I preferred to think had been used only for washing hands and faces. My dad stood awkwardly in the only square foot of floor not occupied by suitcases or boxes.

"All right, you've got everything?" he said.

"I think so," I replied, unable to look him in the eye. I knew his black caterpillar eyebrows were drawn into a continuous questioning line.

"I suppose I'll be off, then, before the traffic gets too bad."

"Okay," I paused. "Shall I come to the car with you?"

"No, no need, you get settled here."

"Okay." My small relief that I wouldn't have to walk back from the car alone with a press of tears behind my eyelids was soon tempered by the realization that this was goodbye.

"Give us a call and let us know how you're doing," he said.

"Will do."

"Love you."

"Love you, too," I said.

And then he was gone.

Sitting on my barely-twin bed, I listened to the excited bustle and chatter of other students moving in, making friends. I'd never quite fit in at high school; my peculiar dedication to academic excellence and rule following had branded me a "swot." I didn't have time for parties, illicit cigarettes behind the bike shed, or dating, which was just as well, because I was never invited. My extracurricular activities were more sedate—playing flute in the orchestra, singing in the school choir, and competing on the swim team. And my singular determination to get into vet school made it easier to ignore the whispered slights in the changing room after PE.

I'd harbored a shy hope that I would finally find my place at university, but not long after my arrival in London it became clear that my state-school education and just-about middle-class upbringing separated me from my classmates, the majority of whom had spent childhoods cantering around country estates while on holiday from private boarding school. I managed to find a small group of friends with backgrounds similar to my own to meet for meals in the dining hall—six girls who also lived in Commonwealth Hall and didn't have pet ponies—but still, my need to spend one more hour revising biochemical pathways set me apart.

Even more alienating than my desire to study hard was my lack of horsemanship. At ten I'd gone through a horse-obsessed phase and had persuaded my parents that riding lessons were a necessary part of my childhood. In jeans and wellies, my sister and I spent every other Saturday morning at the cheaper of the two stables in town, which was more tolerant of our lack of jodhpurs and fancy riding boots.

However, it turned out that I was highly allergic to the beast I'd hoped to feed sugar lumps, and close contact with a horse resulted in instant sneezing and eye swelling. Still, this didn't deter me. I continued taking riding lessons until I could no longer hide my blinding eye irritation from my parents.

Notwithstanding my persistence, I never found equilibrium in the saddle. When my steed went from a trot to a canter, my grip tightened on the reins and my biceps flexed. My white-knuckled hands would rise until they were uselessly hovering in midair, while my feet curled desperately around the stirrups and my frustrated instructor screeched "Keep your hands down!" If I'm honest, I always preferred my Sindy (the UK's more realistic version of Barbie) horse to the real thing. I could plait and style its mane and tail for hours, brushing the man-made fibers until they shone. There was no risk of being stood on or bucked off, and I didn't need to care about my lack of jodhpurs, because Sindy had the perfect outfit, complete with velvet hard hat and riding crop. But at vet school I couldn't avoid horses or the "horsey set" that I'd once so desperately wanted to belong to.

My anatomy dissection class shared one horse—a pony, really— and one cow for the duration of the two-year preclinical course. The first day, they both hung from sturdy hooks through their backs, in disconcerting standing positions. Despite their posture, the nose-numbing tang of formaldehyde and the rubbery grayness of their muscles confirmed their lifelessness. The dissection room was in the basement of the veterinary school, and the only windows were high along one wall, lending a permanent fluorescent-lit austerity to our classes. It was cold and damp, and our white coats did little to protect us. If we didn't roll our sleeves high enough, they slurped up the juices from the stainless steel dissection tables, the cuffs quickly turning a dingy pinkish gray.

In addition to the two large animals at the front of the class, the headless body of a dog or goat lay on each of the tables positioned at precise intervals across the floor. A bucket hung beneath each one under the drain to catch escaping fluids. Trim, muscular ex-racing greyhounds lay stiffly on the cold metal surface, their legs extended and unbending.

There weren't enough dogs to go around. Local shelters wouldn't donate the bodies of euthanized stray dogs for what was considered experimentation, so goats were substituted. Their anatomy was significantly different, but they were of a similar size. We spent painstaking hours in assigned groups of four, dissecting the nerves and blood vessels that were conveniently filled with blue latex for veins and red for arteries. One tiny part of anatomy was assigned each week; for example, the lower, lower half of the foreleg. Clustered around our dripping specimens, intently comparing the precise illustration in *Miller's Dissection of the Dog* to the soggy mess of stringy tissues in front of us, I felt a camaraderie that I hadn't discovered in the university bar. Dissecting the origin and insertion of a leg muscle and teasing apart its innervation was a more comfortable social engagement for me than enjoying a pint in the pub on the way home. Over two years, we gradually whittled down the bodies, with each diminishing carcass carefully restored to its preservative bath at the end of lab every week.

The hours we spent in the cavernous anatomy hall seemed far removed from the consulting room in Hereford and George's warm, cheerful voice. And the cold, set specimens were so separate from the living animals they'd once been that it never crossed my mind to be upset.

That was until one Tuesday afternoon, toward the end of our first year, when we were assigned fresh horse's feet from the local knacker's yard. They had been severed above the fetlock, and the rim of skin and hair still attached to the foot made me wonder what the horse had looked like—an uncomfortable reminder that a short while earlier our specimen had been part of a living body. The flesh was petal pink and the cartilage glistening white, a stark contrast to the colors and textures we usually encountered in anatomy lab.

Despite my unfamiliar proximity to living flesh, foot dissection wasn't bad. The inside of the hoof is secretly beautiful, with tiny pleats that resemble the underside of a mushroom cap perfectly interlinking with matching folds on the pedal bone, almost enough to make you forget the desperate prying needed to separate the two halves.

The knowledge we accumulated of the bones and joints, muscles, tendons, ligaments, and nerves of dogs and cats, goats, sheep, pigs, cows, and horses was tested in a qualifying anatomy examination at the end of our first academic year.

On entering the anatomy lab, we were handed a thin booklet of papers. An overwhelming array of specimens lay before us to be identified, and I barely noticed the now-familiar sour smell. Our anatomy professor stood at the front of the hollow room with a timer linked to a buzzer. He was a tall, slim man with a vertical face, who looked at us through his glasses as if we were samples on a microscope slide.

"Please choose a station and stand next to it," he instructed.

Each table displayed a different-sized morsel of preserved flesh, a foot on one, a forelimb on another. Some had ropey nerves exposed with pieces of string tied around them; others were studded with colored pushpins inserted into a muscle, tendon, or ligament. Each was tagged with a small piece of soggy paper with a number written in black marker.

"Once you have selected a station, please find the corresponding page in your booklet," the professor said. "You will see a question on the table next to the specimen. Please write the answer next to the appropriate number." I glanced down nervously.

"You will have ninety seconds at each station, and the buzzer will sound when it's time to move on to the next." The professor gazed disinterestedly around the room, already looking bored by the prospect of moderating an exam for the next two hours.

"Any questions?" We stayed quiet.

The damp fabric of my shirt caught on my back; the basement room was uncomfortably chilly. I quickly checked my lab coat pocket for the pen I knew was there and moved to the table on my right, where the hind limb of a goat rested. The muscles had been removed, and a piece of grayish string encircled a delicate, white-plastic-looking nerve. The shallow pool of clear liquid surrounding the limb moved determinedly to the edge of the table and the sleeves of my freshly washed lab coat.

The buzzer sounded.

At times during those first two years of veterinary school, when the only living animals I encountered were the fearless, sooty mice who lived between the tracks at the Tube stations, the relevance of the cellular pathways, molecular structures, and biologic mechanisms we studied seemed impossible to realize. And I began to think that I preferred it that way. My lack of horsemanship didn't matter when the only horse I had to handle was fixed in formalin or on the pages of a textbook. The pain, suffering, and distress that disease caused animals were a long way from the frigid dampness of the dissection hall.

But, eventually, after years in the anatomy lab and countless qualifying examinations, it was time to move to the clinical campus in Hertfordshire, a thirty-minute train ride from London. Despite my apprehension about dealing with live patients, it was thrilling to be within sight of the goal I'd set so long ago. My clinical studies lay ahead before I would graduate with a veterinary degree, and I was determined to apply myself with the same commitment I'd given my books. Our stained lab coats were replaced with new, freshly starched ones. The lectures we attended advanced from slides of cells to pictures of the animals they composed. And, finally, we were introduced to the living embodiment of the anatomy, biochemistry, physiology, and pathophysiology we'd spent years studying.

I took to the small animals and their owners, but equine medicine and surgery was still my most dreaded clinical rotation. The patients, and the people who owned them, stirred a deep and uncomfortable confusion within me. My green country wellies, practical in the hospital setting, nevertheless set me apart from the horsey set and their sleek boots with the discreet "Hunter" logo. The university's equine staff were similarly dressed, and significantly more terrifying. There was one particular equine medicine professional who appeared to enjoy making students, interns, residents, and likely other faculty members cry, usually from fear and humiliation. She was the only woman on faculty in the equine department—a hangover from the male dominance of veterinary medicine. Her voice had a gravelly, piercing quality, her confident stride could be heard from twenty paces, and her reputation was fierce.

My clinical duties on the equine rotation required me to jump out of bed at all hours, at the summons of my insistently bleeping pager, and rush to the hospital to "assist" with surgeries or administer medications. Medicating horses can be challenging, especially when you're only half awake. Even instilling eyedrops was nearly impossible—the drops needed to be administered frequently, and a horse's eye is in uncomfortable proximity to its surprisingly sharp teeth. Often we were forced to surgically implant elaborate catheters that tunneled underneath the reluctant horses' strong eyelids to ensure proper application of ocular medications.

The prospect of assisting with a surgery was barely more appealing. Surgery on horses can be difficult, and the risk of the procedure was terrifying. Before the patient arrived on the operating table there was anesthesia to administer. The sight of a sixteen-hand-tall horse crumpling to the ground was amazing, and we nervously hoped that no legs—human or equine—would be broken in the process. We used large padded boxes with mechanized lifting gear to anesthetize and then recover the huge animals. The anesthetists used endotracheal tubes thicker than my forearm to deliver oxygen and anesthetic gases to their enormous patients. Once the horses were asleep we would shackle and attach them to the overhead winch that lifted them into the operating theater. It could take a frenetic hour to get a horse anesthetized and delivered safely to the surgical table.

Horses are not designed to lie in one place for long periods. Blood supply and oxygen delivery to vital areas becomes quickly compromised in recumbent horses due to their large muscle mass and dense skeletons. Additionally, the weight of their organs can cause lung collapse after an hour or two under anesthesia. Every surgery was a race against the clock, since we knew that the longer it took, the more likely it was that the horse wouldn't get up. My role during surgery was narrowly defined. Occasionally I would be asked to hand over an instrument or hold suction equipment, but generally these minor tasks were considered by some too expert. Consequently, standing still—not touching or breathing on the sterile field—was the typical extent of my duties.

However, I assumed it was unlikely that I would ever touch a horse in a medical capacity beyond my veterinary education. My passion did not lie in the surgical excavation of my patient's tissues, and the diagnosis and treatment of disease in cats and dogs was further advanced than in large-animal medicine. This, combined with my ambivalence toward my larger patients, made it clear that my post-graduation interactions with hooved beasts would be limited. I knew that my future lay in small-animal medicine. I squirreled the information about equine, bovine, ovine, and porcine medicine away, tucking it into the sulci of my hippocampus, where it slowly faded, along with many of my memories of my years at veterinary school. There were some moments, though, that stayed with me long after my need for them had expired.

"You remember what you're going to do?" Peter asked.

"Yes," I answered, hoping he'd repeat the directions one last time.

"You are going to draw an imaginary line from one ear to the opposite eye, and then repeat for the other ear and eye. The two lines will make an X. The spot where the lines cross is where you will place the gun. It's going to be higher up than you think; remember that."

I nodded.

"Tell me what you're going to do next," he said.

"I'm going to position the gun's muzzle flat against the horse's head, at the same angle as the neck to the ground so the bullet goes directly into the cerebrum and cerebellum rather than across the top of the forehead."

"All right, good. Now once you've got the positioning right, remember that you want to squeeze the trigger gently; don't jab at it with your finger, and whatever you do don't step backward at the last moment. And don't close your eyes. You're only going to get one shot. It needs to be done right. We don't want this horse to suffer."

My anxiety ratcheted up. I was being entrusted with a huge responsibility, and whatever I did, I didn't want to mess it up. I pictured myself firmly gripping the lead rope attached to the head collar. I silently recited a mantra: *I will not close my eyes. I will not close my eyes. I will not close my eyes.*

Peter loaded the gun, keeping the safety on, and we walked across the field. It wasn't difficult to catch the pony. She was used to people, and we must have seemed like friendly visitors. We led her to the flattest part of the field, not far from the road. A scrubby hedge only partially blocked the view of passing traffic. My hands were shaking. I took the gun. I wanted to give it back, but I knew I would not. Peter stood several feet behind me.

I reached up and gently patted the pony on her forehead. Up close I could see the sharp bones of her pelvis pushing against her skin. Brushing aside her wiry forelock, I silently calculated where to place my shot. Her gray hair softly bristled under my sweaty palm. I could smell her sweet, grassy horsiness.

I gripped the gun in my left hand and raised it to the spot on her forehead. It felt heavier and denser than I'd imagined. I'd seen guns only in movies, being waved around with relaxed nonchalance. With my right hand I grasped the lead rope. Placing the pistol to her head helped steady my hand. Her gaze was level with mine, and for a moment I stared into the black-brown liquid of her eyes.

I had one shot to get it right.

The sound ricocheted and reverberated off the trees that lined the road. Obliterating and unmistakably metallic, it bounced and spun inside my head. I could hear nothing else. Where, a second ago, there had been a smallish gray pony, now there was just a field. I looked down, and there she was, her eyes open but flat. There was a perfectly round, dark hole in the middle of the imaginary cross on her forehead with red-black blood oozing out. I took my stethoscope out of my pocket and attempted to find her heart. My ears still deadened, I wondered if I would hear the slow thirty beats a minute even if a pulse was there. The noise and weight of my perfect shot lingered long after her last breath.

I handed the gun to Peter, my hands still shaking, and we walked back to the car to drive to our next call. The knacker's van would pull in shortly to pick up the body.

"Well done," Peter said.

"Thanks."

"Did you keep your eyes open?" he asked.

"Yes," I lied.

# CHAPTER TWO

# Hercules

I n the middle of June 2000, I arrived in the United States with two suitcases, the promise of a rotating internship in small-animal medicine and surgery, and a J-1 visa. It was a month before I would technically graduate from veterinary school, and four days before I would discover if I'd passed my final exams and qualify as a veterinarian. Had I failed, my suitcases, visa, and I would've been on the next plane home.

My first taste of American veterinary medicine had come during my penultimate year of college, when I spent a six-week externship at Cornell University, where the array of diagnostic tests available—and the lunch options at the snack cart—seemed limitless. The small-animal hospital at the Royal Veterinary College is considered among the best in the United Kingdom, but it seemed modest and quaint compared to the caseload and facilities at Cornell. George, Peter, and the clinic I'd grown up in seemed like they were from a different century. I had a sense before my trip to Cornell that I wanted to pursue academic medicine after graduation. The idea of stepping into a practice straight out of school was unappealing, and I hadn't outgrown my passion for studying. The two weeks I'd spent on the internal medicine rotation at Cornell had opened my eyes to the possibility of a career in small-animal internal medicine.

Once I set my sights on my post-graduation goal I did everything in my power to achieve it, in the same way that I'd steadfastly pursued getting into and then through veterinary school. But when I realized that the opportunities to pursue specialized training in the United Kingdom were limited, I didn't hesitate to apply for an internship in the States. Moving across the ocean to gain more advanced training didn't feel like a decision; it was merely the next step on the path to achieving my goal. My time at university had already distanced me from my family, especially during the clinical years, when weekends were spent on call, and vacations were spent seeing practice. The small group of friends I'd established at vet school, and the boyfriend I'd started dating a few months before my departure, were no rival for my singular determination. It wasn't until I stepped onto the plane at Heathrow that I could see everything and everyone I was leaving behind.

The only things waiting for me in Philadelphia were the promise of an internship at the University of Pennsylvania and a room in an apartment I would share with two fellow interns. The apartment was on the second floor of a battered two-story house a five-minute walk from the University of Pennsylvania's veterinary teaching hospital (VHUP) in West Philadelphia. And along with Dave and Chris—the intern mates I had yet to meet—I would also be sharing the apartment with their pets; a Doberman pinscher, a German shepherd, and several cats. It would be the first time I'd lived with the animals I'd studied.

The social hierarchy of my new living arrangement was established as quickly as introductions were made. Dave, who had secured the apartment, was the only U.S. citizen and was a good ten years older than Chris and me. He requisitioned the largest and best-appointed room with a bay window that looked out over a street of parked cars, occasional drug deals, and trash. Not exactly great, but compared to my tiny room with a view of the neighbor's brick wall, which I could reach out and touch, it seemed luxurious.

Dave owned Max, the German shepherd, and three cats—who remained sequestered in Dave's room. Max was middle-aged and had a graying muzzle that matched Dave's receding hairline and increasingly accentuated widow's peak. Their deep, tangible bond was obvious, and reflected in Max's intense stare whenever Dave was in the room. Max spent his days either tightly curled under Dave's desk in the hospital's closet-like intern office or lounging in Dave's bedroom. Max was a one-man dog, and Dave was a man's man. Max would give me a cursory acknowledgment when I can home, a half-raised eyebrow if I addressed him directly, and a stubborn reluctance if I suggested a walk when Dave was stuck at the hospital. I suspected that his ambivalence toward me was a reflection of his owner's feelings. It wasn't that Dave wasn't friendly, but I, once again, didn't fit in. Chris and Dave were gracious enough housemates, including me on trips to Ikea to furnish our apartment and to the grocery store to stock my designated cupboard with peculiar foods that looked familiar but proved unsavory. But the beer-drinking, hockey-watching camaraderie immediately established between Dave and Chris was a club, and I wasn't a member.

Chris was Canadian, and had rescued his young Doberman, Tye, from his vet school on Prince Edward Island. Chris's red hair and beard (which he'd grow to a wild length during our internship) seemed to complement Tye's liver-and-tan coat, and they shared an untamed energy. Tye was barely contained by the crate where he spent twelve or more hours a day while Chris was at the hospital, equally desperate to get out of his white coat. They, too, were a long way from home. Chris showed me pictures of his vet school lodgings—a solitary, dark wooden house, surrounded by the sprawling greenness of woods and fields with no buildings or roads in

sight. It seemed a more appropriate setting for Chris and his rambunctious young dog than West Philadelphia, where the local park
was best known for drugs and prostitution.

I was assigned the smallest bedroom, an afterthought of a room
so tiny that it would've been impossible to swing a cat once my bed
was moved in. The unofficial residents of the house included mice,
rats, squirrels, and various decades-old mold spores. At first I didn't
believe Dave when he told me the fingertip-size dent in the neighbor's door was from a bullet, but after my first week in West Philadelphia, I did.

At the start of my internship, I'd sit on my new Ikea bed in my
new apartment, surrounded by an unfamiliar city, and wonder what
I was doing. Every morning, I'd grab the portable phone from the
kitchen, the black plastic slick against my palm, take it to my bedroom, and attempt to call home. The long numeric sequence of
country code, area code, and then my home number was difficult to
dial. The familiar double ring when the line connected was soothing—
until it gave way to the hollow persistence of an unanswered phone.
Even if I could get the sequence right, the time difference meant that
everyone was at work when I called.

I'd hang up and search my address book for the number of one of
my vet school friends, but my certainty that their new practices kept
them busy and happy stayed my hand. I pictured them seeing patients, driving to large-animal calls, or chatting with colleagues about
cases over a midmorning cup of tea. The familiarity I imagined them
feeling, in spite of the novelty of a new practice, widened the distance between us, expanding the Atlantic Ocean from my phone to
theirs.

In the first month of my internship I was assigned to emergency
days, a grueling schedule of 7 A.M. to 7 P.M., otherwise known as "bap-
tism by fire." The fifteen- to sixteen-hour days I spent in the hospital
left little time to worry about the social limitations of my living situation. Everything was suddenly different. The drug names I'd
crammed into my head during vet school were now meaningless; I

had to learn an alien language of U.S. names for drugs, along with entirely new units and reference ranges that clouded my understanding of normal and abnormal—the metric system replaced by strangely archaic ounces, pounds, inches, and feet.

The majority of the drug inventory available at the Veterinary Hospital of the University of Pennsylvania was formulated for human, rather than animal, consumption, a fact I hadn't realized until I was the one writing the prescriptions. And, as such, concentrations of liquid medications, tablet sizes, and the amount of injectable drug contained in a vial were often inconvenient.

In school, I'd assumed that the medications discussed in lectures and used in clinics were made for the animals we treated. In practice, veterinary equivalents of the medications we used were unavailable. From insulin to antibiotics to narcotics, everything was labeled "For Human Use Only."

The emergency room was the largest space dedicated to the care of small animals I'd seen, at least six times bigger than George's consulting room back in England. There were three waist-high stainless steel tables for the triage, stabilization, and treatment of cats and dogs in the center of the room. One had a deep bath-like sink with a grate on top for "dirty" procedures such as clipping and cleaning wounds. Two large oxygen cages were stacked against one wall for animals with difficulty breathing—usually cats with asthma or dogs in heart failure, but once an albino boa constrictor with pneumonia. A small bank of cages off the central area housed patients who needed to stay for observation or further treatment. Big dogs too sick to be mobile—often those hit by a car—lay on blankets on the floor, where they could be easily monitored. The wall opposite the oxygen cages was lined with a bank of cheery blue-green cabinets and a work surface for processing lab samples, laying out supplies, and writing up treatment sheets. The long bench was crowded with baskets of different-sized intravenous catheters, syringes, needles, blood tubes, and the other equipment needed to stabilize a crashing patient. I'd never seen so much veterinary stuff shuffled into such a tight space—not even in the boot of Peter's SUV.

There were no windows, and the only way to determine the passage of time was the clock above the doctors' station, which was a small nook for writing up records, grabbing a quick snack, and every so often sitting down. A dense forest of rainbow-hued paper fanned out from file folders on the wall, each color allotted a specific role—golden yellow transfer sheets, pink treatment sheets, baby blue bloodwork requisition forms. It was a straightforward system, but overwhelming until memorized.

The floor was industrial-strength linoleum that was always halfway between clean and dirty. Large puddles of blood, urine, diarrhea, or vomit were cleaned immediately, but smaller splashes were often forgotten in the hubbub of stabilizing a critical patient. Animal hair was everywhere, and it remained tucked into the corners of the room despite our efforts to clean it up.

The patients of the preceding few hours determined the smell of the emergency room. I learned the shockingly pungent, eye-watering distinction between urine from intact versus neutered cats. And I became adept at identifying the particular odor of bloody diarrhea caused by canine parvovirus.

I also learned a fundamental lesson not taught in any lecture: Listen to the technicians. Those who'd worked in the emergency room for years saved me on a daily basis. Their seasoned suggestions of a test to run or a medication to administer were invaluable to a clueless intern. The glaring inexperience of my first days as a veterinarian was nothing new to the team of senior doctors, residents, and technicians; a fresh class of interns stood blinking in the fluorescent harshness of the ER every June.

From the first day of orientation my position as an intern was firmly established. Interns ranked marginally above the students, but below almost every member of the veterinary staff. My hard-won title, *veterinarian,* meant little to the technicians, and less to the most senior veterinary specialists who headed up the clinical departments. If my name had not been embroidered on my white coat I am certain some faculty members would have called me "You!" for the entire year.

The residents were positioned between the interns and faculty. VHUP residencies typically lasted three years, and every clinical department from dentistry to surgery trained residents. The number for each specialty was based on the size of the department and their caseload. Internal medicine had four residents each year, while smaller services such as dermatology would take one every two or three years.

Internship success depended on getting along with the residents, second only to winning over the technicians. In many ways the residents ran the hospital. Regardless of specialty, they saw the most cases, worked the longest hours, and were the people to call if you had a problem patient. They usually remembered what it was like to be an intern, which meant that they were willing to lend a sympathetic ear, or hand, when things became overwhelming. The residents were my heroes, more accessible than the god-like senior clinicians, and close enough that I could imagine myself in their position.

I was still a year away from residency, but only a month or two separated me from the students I taught and supervised. The different structure of veterinary training in the United Kingdom meant that, at twenty-five, I was younger than most of the final-year students. And the bewildering adjustment to a new country made me feel even more immature. The novelty of my English accent muted some of the potential conflict between me, a naïve young intern, and the students who were paying close to $50,000 a year for enrollment at the University of Pennsylvania.

I understood the awkwardness of my position. When I was a student a few months earlier, I'd found the interns both helpful and confusingly annoying. Sometimes they were competition for performing basic procedures, a source of constant irritation when students were desperately wanting to try out new clinical skills. But interns were also good company on overnight ICU shifts, in which hours were occupied debating critical questions such as how hungry we'd have to be to eat cat food.

In the everyday high-paced bustle of VHUP it was easy to forget that we'd all—interns and residents—made a voluntary choice to be there. Unlike in human medicine, veterinary internships and residencies aren't mandatory. Upon graduation I was free to practice medicine and perform surgery on any species, and I was one of only two in my class of almost one hundred who'd pursued an internship straight out of school.

I was lucky: I landed a coveted position at a highly regarded academic institution, which would pave the way for my future in veterinary medicine. I didn't appreciate, at the time, how significant my year at the University of Pennsylvania would prove to be. I was solely focused on my overwhelming goal of survival—for my patients and myself.

Like all VHUP interns, I was assigned to a clinical service in the hospital, and every month I would rotate to a different department. I was always a week away from finding my feet on shifting ground; by the time I was comfortable in a particular department it was time to switch, and the responsibilities, caseloads, and expectations were different on every service.

During my first month, in the emergency room, I was left to my own devices between eight and nine each morning, when the senior doctors attended resident teaching rounds. I was the only qualified veterinarian in the ER for that excruciating hour, and my responsibilities included triaging and admitting new cases, and keeping an eye on the day's ER patients. I spent most of that time hovering in the middle of the treatment area, silently praying for no new patient arrivals. My primary goal for the hour was to avoid anything remotely resembling the practice of veterinary medicine, and, when that wasn't possible, to avoid killing anything. *First do no harm* was illuminated in neon, flashing in my head.

On a Tuesday morning in late June, the senior clinicians had left the emergency room. The bank of cages was gradually emptying of patients being transferred to their respective specialty services— orthopedics for broken legs, soft tissue surgery for abdominal masses and intestinal obstructions, and internal medicine for everything else. Residents came and went, leaving students and interns to transport patients out of the ER, along the corridor to the elevator, and up three floors to the wards. The sea of still-unfamiliar faces did little to calm my rising nerves.

I peered into the oxygen cage trying to determine if the dyspneic cat's breathing had changed in the thirty seconds since I'd last checked. The cat's coat was dull and spiky. She had not been grooming herself, and I had an urge to smooth her rumpled fur, to calm her jagged breathing with my touch, but I knew that by opening the cage I'd only make her worse. One of the technicians, Elisa, entered the emergency room. She was a few years older than me and was considered one of the more senior and experienced staff members. I felt wary of her. I had the distinct feeling that she was waiting for me to slip up.

"There's a GSW coming in," she said. "The police department called; they're bringing it in. ETA ten minutes."

*GSW?* I didn't want to betray my ignorance, having already been caught out by HBC, hit by car, which we'd called a road traffic accident, or RTA, in England.

"It's a big dog," she continued. "Got in the way of crossfire. It sounds pretty bad, shot in the chest."

I suddenly realized GSW meant gunshot wound. I looked at the clock and caught my breath—ten past eight—fifty minutes before the senior clinicians would arrive. Then I looked at Elisa. She was petite, pretty, always wore makeup, and managed to keep a manicure look-

ing fresh all week. Her neat, brightly colored scrubs made me feel
baggy and crumpled.

"You're joking, right? I mean, dogs don't get shot." I laughed, sure
that she was testing me, hazing the new intern. I'd almost fallen for
it, too.

Elisa looked at me. She wasn't smiling.

"No I'm not," she said. "The dog will be here in ten minutes.
What do you want set up?"

I had absolutely no idea what to do with a dog who'd been shot,
or how to get back onto Elisa's good side. This definitely hadn't been
covered at vet school.

"Sorry," I said. "It's just, we don't really have guns in England, and
I didn't think a dog could be shot. Sorry."

"We see them pretty often here, so you better get used to it," Elisa
replied.

"Great, yes. It's good to see new things. What do you think we'll
need?"

I could only hope she'd come through. I relied on my plastered-on
smile to hide the redness rising to my cheeks, and my white coat to
hide the rapidly expanding rings of sweat under my arms.

"Well . . ." she said.

I smiled harder, looked at the clock: eight-sixteen; the dog would
arrive in less than five minutes.

"Maybe we could set up for an IV catheter and hang a liter of fluids?" I said.

"Right," Elisa said. "Do you want me to set up for a chest tap,
too?" She'd thrown me a lifeline.

Chest tap? That meant I would be sticking a large needle between
the dog's ribs to drain blood from the thoracic cavity, or air if the bullet had gone into the lung. I'd seen it done, and I'd assisted a few
times, but to do one by myself, with no other doctors around . . . I
tried to remember the landmarks, what I would need to do, which rib
space, how high up the chest wall to pass the needle. Elisa stared at
me expectantly.

"Yes, that's a good idea," I said. "Hopefully, we won't need it."

While I was recalibrating my expectations for the next forty minutes, the page came in.

"Triage to the front with a gurney. Stat."

Two assistants headed for the door of the emergency room grabbing towels and a gurney. I walked to the crash table where my new patient would land, my legs trembling. The edge of the stainless steel was fringed with lengths of white tape ready to secure an intravenous catheter. Gauze squares soaked in dilute chlorhexidine scrub solution and alcohol sat in two small paper party bowls, ready for use.

Elisa finished setting up the chest tap and looked at me. "What size gloves are you?"

"Uh . . . small?"

"How about six and a half?" she asked.

I had the fleeting thought that no one at home was going to believe I was treating a dog with a GSW. Then the door of the emergency room glided open and a broad policeman, with—I couldn't help noticing and then was unable to ignore—a gun strapped to his belt, bundled a large black dog through it.

"Over here," shouted Elisa. And the policeman dumped the dog onto the table in front of me.

I looked down at my patient and noticed a smear of blood on the table, but I couldn't see where it was coming from. The dog's black coat hid the spot where the skin and muscle had been breached. He looked calm. His head was up and he seemed curious about the hospital, his personality intact despite the hole in his chest wall.

"What's his name?" I asked.

"Hercules, I think," replied the police officer.

"Where's his owner?" Elisa cut in.

"He's coming," the officer replied. "He doesn't have transport, so he's coming by bus. Should be here in a half hour or so." The officer seemed unconcerned.

"In half an hour this dog could be dead," said Elisa.

I turned to Elisa. "What should we do?" Hercules was now my

patient, and it was my job to save him. He was a young, handsome Doberman; the tan markings on his face were sharp against his black fur. His coat was shiny, his ears still puppyish and floppy. The two tan spots above the corner of each eye made it look like he was about to ask me a question.

"Not much, without the owner's permission," Elisa replied. "But if you think his condition is life-threatening, we can administer emergency care to stabilize him."

I looked at Hercules. His breathing was ragged. The motion of his rib cage was exaggerated and irregular, each arc of bone distinct beneath his taut black skin. I cautiously pulled up his lip to look at his gums. His muzzle was downy and warm; I noted each of his black whiskers, the juvenile whiteness of his teeth, the weight of his head rested in my palm. His gums were pale—washed out rather than vibrant pink. He was bleeding more than the smear of blood on the table revealed. I needed to make a decision. Did I begin treatment without owner consent? Or did I wait for the owner to arrive, only for it to be too late when we finally obtained approval?

"TPR?" I asked.

"Temp 100.8, heart rate 180, resps 54."

His heart and respiratory rates were way too high. Was he in pain from the wound, or was he bleeding into his chest?

"Okay," I said. "Let's get a front leg catheter in. What's his weight?"

"I'd guess about one hundred pounds," Elisa replied. "We're not getting him on the scale right now."

I pulled my calculator from my pocket to work out his body weight in kilos, trying to remember the conversion formula to calculate his shock fluid dose.

"Do you want to bolus a liter?" Elisa suggested.

I paused, the calculator gripped in my right hand. Hercules was losing blood, and I didn't want to lose all credibility.

"Sure," I said. "A liter."

"How do his lungs sound?" Elisa asked.

I grabbed my stethoscope and hastily shoved the two small black mushrooms into my ears. I hoped Hercules's heart and lung sounds would drown out the doubt in my head. How had I not listened to his chest yet?

I auscultated his heart first—hearing the crinkling rustle of his fur against my stethoscope every time he inhaled. There are subtleties in the way a heart sounds that can be detected only when you've listened to hundreds, if not thousands, of them. Hercules's heart rate was too high, but I needed to determine if it sounded dull, which would suggest that fluid was building up in his thoracic cavity, in the space his lungs should occupy, or in the pericardial sac surrounding his heart. Was there an abnormal rhythm, suggesting damage to the heart muscle, detectable in the rapid hammering? It was my call. I listened to both sides of his chest. I wanted to be thorough, but I was also buying time. My next decisions could mean life or death for Hercules.

I looked up from his black flank. "Let's get an ECG and blood pressure," I said. "Also, let's pull for a CBC, chemistry panel, blood gas, PCV, and total solids and coagulation test."

"Do you want a lactate with that, too?" Elisa asked.

"Yes, please."

"We've pulled the blood already," Elisa replied. I hadn't noticed, but when I looked down the darkly filled blue, purple, and red-topped tubes were lined on the tabletop.

"Let's run the PCV and blood gas first and send the rest to the lab," I said.

The liter of fluids dashed into Hercules's intravenous catheter; the bag was almost finished. I checked his gums again. Still light pink. Felt his pulse. Not as strong. Hercules's head rested on the table, his nose and front paws dangling off the edge. His claws were shiny in the overhead light, as if he'd had a pedicure on the way to the hospital, each nail completely black against the rich burnished tan of his feet and legs. I wanted to hold his paw, feel its weight and warmth, but I resisted, knowing it would comfort me more than him. I cautiously looked at the right side of Hercules's rib cage. The lower part of his thorax lay flat against the table, but I could see that a small patch of his dark coat was stickily clumped and wet about halfway up his chest, behind his front leg. I touched the area, and when I pulled my fingers back, they were covered in blood. Hercules turned his head sharply, shooting me an accusatory look. I petted his snout, an apology for the pain I'd caused and the pain that was still to come.

"Let's clip this area here." I gestured to where I'd touched. "I think that might be the bullet wound."

"Is there an exit wound?" asked Elisa.

"A what?"

"Usually if there's an entry wound there's another place where the bullet leaves. If not, that could be really bad; means he'll need surgery."

I looked again at his chest. A bullet was so outside my frame of reference I hadn't considered that it might still be inside Hercules.

"I don't see one," I replied, but I didn't know what I was looking for, or its likely location. I had a vague sense that a bullet's trajectory depended on where it was shot from. My experience with guns was confined to a horse in a Herefordshire field.

I looked at the clock. It was still half an hour until help arrived. I was on my own. I calculated what I knew: Hercules had been shot; it looked like he was bleeding, probably into his chest; his breathing was irregular and had not improved despite the liter of fluids he'd received. It didn't look good. I worried that he had an ongoing bleed into his chest, which meant the bullet had hit a major blood vessel or lacerated his lung. In either case, he was going to need surgery, fast, if we were going to save him.

Elisa began trimming the fur from the area of the suspected bullet wound, and the buzz of the clippers startled me into action. An assistant cradled Hercules's head in the crook of her arm, holding him tight against her chest, as if shielding a child from the pain of an injection. The clipper blades were smeared with blood and small clumps of dark, matted hair. Beneath, an innocuous-looking pink hole about the size of a penny was exposed. It didn't fit. The consequences seemed too brutal for this little mouth of tissue. It looked like his body was already trying to seal itself shut and forget what had happened. The size of the hole made me want to believe that things weren't so bad, but the tracing on the electrocardiogram made me change my mind. The ragged green line scuttling across the screen showed that every ten to fifteen beats there was an ugly, abnormal complex, which meant that Hercules's heart was irritated, either from being grazed by the bullet or from blood loss and lack of oxygen. The machine sounded an alarm every time his heart rate exceeded the normal parameters set, and my own pulse raced to keep time.

"Let's get him to X-ray," I said. "We need to get a better look at what's going on."

"Do you think he's stable enough to move?" Elisa asked.

"I'm not sure," I replied. "We need to be quick, but I don't know how else to figure out the damage and what we need to do. We'll gurney him down and take a DV, not a VD, so he doesn't have to lie on his back. Let's take oxygen with us, too. I don't like how he's breathing."

"What about his fluids?" another technician asked.

I resisted the urge to pull out my calculator; instead I clutched it through my coat pocket and hoped for the right calculation by osmosis.

"What's his PCV and total solids?" I asked.

"PCV twenty-five percent, total solids five."

He was bleeding—the values were too low. Hercules needed a blood transfusion. His chest moved forcefully and he released a small shrug of a grunt on each exhale. He occasionally shifted his weight to a more comfortable position, but otherwise he'd become worryingly still.

"Let's take the fluids with us," I said. "We'll give another liter and then recheck his PCV and total solids. Can we get a blood type?"

"There should be enough sample left," the assistant said. "Do you want me to add that on at the lab?"

"Yes, please. And we need to put a stat on that; I think he's going to need some packed cells soon."

In a tangle of wires, IV lines, and oxygen hoses we moved Hercules from the table to a gurney, but his long legs were folded awkwardly and the ECG leads caught below his body, stretching and pulling at the machine. I didn't want to lose the security of the green line tracing across the screen, but the ECG couldn't go with us. I could rely on my fingers to feel his pulse and my ears to listen to his heart. We disconnected the leads and tugged them out from underneath him.

I didn't want Hercules to break the hospital maxim *Nothing dies in radiology*. I had to get him down the corridor and onto the X-ray table, get the X-rays taken, then get him back onto the gurney and returned to the relative safety of the emergency room as quickly as possible. Hercules rested precariously on the gurney; the blue straps we'd Velcroed loosely over his body looked too flimsy to hold him.

Even though Hercules's X-rays could be taken in a millisecond, positioning him appropriately without human restraint was a significant challenge. In order to examine his lungs, he needed to lie on his side on the radiology table with his front legs extended far enough forward that they would not overlie his chest, while also keeping perfectly still. Sandbags, bolsters, and other props could be used to keep him in place, but relying on these to restrain a large, struggling dog could prove particularly challenging. The alternative, of putting ourselves in line of the beam, even protected with lead-lined attire, was strongly discouraged due to the risk from repeated X-ray exposure.

Once Hercules was positioned, the X-ray beam had to be collimated to the desired area, the plate positioned, and the exposure set based on his size. For Hercules, laboring to breathe and in pain, any one of these could be the critical step too far. For him, the danger was not the flash of X-ray exposure, but rather the preparation to obtain the image.

In veterinary medicine, radiographs are widely employed as a first-line diagnostic for such diverse problems as limping, coughing, and vomiting. They add an essential dimension to our ability to investigate illness in patients who cannot verbally communicate. The results can be instantly revelatory and even illuminate the things our pets get up to while we're out—a black-and-white universe of trash cans plundered, sock drawers ransacked, and treasures long forgotten under the couch. For Hercules, I was going to use radiographs to determine if the bullet was still in his chest, and the location and extent of the damage, which was vital information we could then use to formulate a plan—as long as he didn't die in the process.

We maneuvered out of the emergency room to make the sharp left into radiology. Hercules was sprawled on the gurney, his back legs curled to the side and his feet brushing the doorframe. I looked down the corridor and noted a tall male figure approaching. I was relieved by the sight of another veterinarian. He looked experienced, I didn't recognize him as an intern, and he was wearing a long white coat, indicating that his rank was above that of a student. When we got closer I saw that he was smiling, and, despite his quick stride, he had a calm stillness about him.

"Hi, Matt!" Elisa exclaimed, suddenly alert and attentive.

"Hey, what's up?" Matt turned to include me.

"Hi." I wasn't sure if my blush was from relief or embarrassment.

Elisa jumped in, "We're trying to get this dog to radiology. He's been shot. Cool case, huh?"

I hoped she didn't feel the pulse of anger I aimed at her when she usurped me.

"D'you think he's going to need surgery?" Matt asked.

So far my plan for Hercules hadn't extended much beyond the radiology department. But I realized that by placing an intravenous catheter, giving fluids, and initiating all the other steps I'd taken in the past half hour, I'd started a sequence of events that was bigger than any of those small actions. I had decided to treat Hercules without his owner's permission, and I now had to follow that decision through.

"Maybe?" I replied. I was trying to guess who Matt was, and frantically calculating whether I should ask him for help. "I'm not sure what's going on, but I think he's bleeding into his chest. He's not breathing well, and he has an arrhythmia." I glanced at my patient barely balanced on the gurney. "We were on our way to get chest rads." I wanted to keep moving, to return Hercules to the relatively familiar safety of the emergency room, but no one else seemed to share my concern.

"I'm Matt Thomas, a surgery resident." He extended his hand. "I don't think we've met."

"I'm Suzy," I replied, trying to mirror his nonchalance. Maybe I was overreacting; maybe my anxiety was due to my inexperience and not my patient's condition. "I'm a new intern. I've never seen a gunshot before."

"You can't have been in Philly long, then," Matt replied. Elisa nodded, I assumed at my naïveté.

"No," I said. "People don't shoot dogs in England." I turned to look at Hercules again, hiding my embarrassment in solicitude for my patient. His breathing seemed even more labored than it had a few minutes earlier. I moved to the front of the gurney, hoping to indicate the level of urgency I was feeling.

"Is there anything I can do to help?" Matt asked, still smiling. He looked at Hercules. "Looks like we need to get this guy to radiology and back fast. Don't want him dying while he's down there."

I nodded. "If you're not too busy, that would be great." We began slowly moving down the corridor again, the weight of Hercules on the gurney taking a moment to catch up with our effort.

"I'm going to page surgery and let them know this one might be coming up; he's not looking so good," Matt said. I nodded again, relieved that my concern was justified.

"Is the owner on board?" Matt asked.

The owner. I'd almost forgotten about him.

"He's not here yet," I said. He was still nameless and faceless. All I knew was that he had a dog named Hercules. "I'm sure he'd want us to do everything we can." I sounded more certain than I felt. I had no idea if what I'd said was true. I felt dangerously out of my depth. The implications of owner consent, payment for services, and the sometimes-testy relationship between veterinarians, their patients, and their clients was far off and peripheral in this overwhelming sea of newness.

"We can figure that out later," Matt said. "Right now, let's find out what's going on with this dog."

We formed a shambling procession to radiology, Elisa edging closer to Matt in the crowd, subtly shifting her attention from our patient to the new surgery resident.

The gurney was almost too wide to fit through the door to the X-ray room, and it took more than one try to maneuver it through the space. Our arrival had done nothing to ease my tension. The X-ray technicians were fierce when it came to positioning patients correctly for radiographs and enforcing proper safety regulations. I had to watch Hercules from a small lead-lined box in the corner of the room while the technicians expertly arranged his limbs to get the best shot. Hercules was reluctant to extend his right front leg, likely due to the discomfort of the bullet wound on that side.

"Has he had any pain medications?" Matt, standing next to me, asked.

Pain meds? I'd forgotten that my patient was in pain during my effort to save his life.

"No," I replied.

"Let's see how this goes," Matt replied. "But if he keeps struggling you might want to run and grab some hydro from the ER."

"Right," I replied. I added pain control to my silent inventory of mistakes I'd made with Hercules. Running back to the emergency room and hiding under the doctor's desk was an option I considered, but, with gentle persuasion, Hercules lay still long enough to take the X-rays.

The radiographs revealed that Hercules had blood in his chest and a bullet lodged in his lung. He needed surgery to remove the entire affected lung lobe and control the bleeding, and then an ICU stay with chest tubes, oxygen supplementation, an arterial line to monitor his blood pressure, and a jugular catheter for continuous venous access. The cost of his care would run into the thousands, and I hadn't spoken to the person responsible for the bill. We were still waiting for his bus to arrive.

Hercules's case was gaining momentum. Each new finding led to a necessary treatment. His blood pressure told us he needed more fluids and blood products. His ECG told us he needed medication to stabilize his heart rhythm. Matt's unbridled excitement at the prospect of an emergency thoracotomy on an otherwise slow Tuesday morning was evident when he hurried off to find the rest of the surgical team and alert the anesthesia staff. But I was increasingly struggling to identify the line between what needed to be done immediately and what could wait until I talked to the owner. Could Hercules go to surgery without his owner's consent? I didn't know the answer, and Matt was gone before I could ask.

Despite the commotion around him, Hercules lay quietly on the ER table. He seemed smaller somehow—less animate than when he'd arrived. I called his name, trying to convince myself that he was bored or scared, but he didn't lift his head, or even an eyebrow. It seemed that he had only enough energy to breathe, and even that was becoming exhausting.

While I wrangled the needs of my patient and waited for his owner, the surgical team arrived. Surgeons in vet hospitals move in packs—a many-limbed, multi-headed beast that is difficult to stop once it gets moving. Even so, I was frustrated to be relegated to the back row of the gallery forming around my patient while Elisa stood resolutely at Hercules's side. She was the smallest person in the group, but her rank and experience positioned her centrally. She was an accepted member of the hospital staff, her presence expected, while my stature was unproven and tentative.

"Whose case is this?" asked one of the older-looking vets, glancing around. I didn't know who he was.

"Mine?" I said, half-raising my hand. I was about to be grilled on Hercules's blood gas values, PCV and total solids, and every other parameter that had instantly evaporated from my memory. At that moment one of the receptionists appeared to inform me that Hercules's owner, a Mr. Brown, had arrived.

"Should I go and talk to him?" I asked the crowd, directing my question toward Matt, the one face I recognized. His posture had changed now that his superiors surrounded him. He'd become intent and serious.

"Someone needs to, don't they?" replied the older surgeon. "And it's not going to be me, so you need to go get permission for us to take this dog to surgery. Now."

I hesitated. I knew the owner didn't really have a choice; the options were surgery or euthanasia. Hercules wouldn't make it on his own. I was reluctant to leave my patient, but my job was to get him to surgery and then remain in the emergency room to treat whatever came through the door next. Hercules's life was no longer in my hands. Ignoring the senior surgeon's urgency, I moved to Hercules's head, afraid he might not be there when I got back. I was compelled to run my hand down the fantastic softness of his ear. I lingered at his side for a second before rushing off to find his owner. On my way I glanced at the box on the wall where the new patients' charts waited. There were already three metal files sitting expectantly in the bin. I had another ten hours of emergencies to go.

I stepped uncertainly into the small, suddenly too-warm consulting room and positioned myself behind the flat expanse of the exam table. Hercules's owner sat uncomfortably in a plastic chair pushed against the opposite wall. He was wearing the clothes and bewilderment of someone whose plans had suddenly and irrevocably been changed. His dingy undershirt and loose, crumpled pants suggested a day of lazing around the house in the sluggish air of a box fan ill-matched to the humid Philadelphia summer. He was an older man; gray-white stubble dirtied his face, and a wrinkled, confused frown grazed his forehead. I stood straight and attempted a reassuring smile.

I placed my hands on the table in front of me. The cool steel surface was comforting until I saw the two sweaty handprints that betrayed me when I anxiously shoved my hands back in my pockets.

"Are you the doctor?" he asked.

I forced my smile. "Yes, I'm Dr. Suzy Fincham. I'm taking care of Hercules."

"Jeez, they make 'em young these days. Shouldn't you be in school? Where is he, anyway? He's not dead, is he? He's all I've got."

"Mr. Brown." I swallowed to keep the rising tremor from my voice. "Mr. Brown, Hercules is alive, but he's a very sick dog. He's been shot in the chest, and the bullet appears to be lodged in his lung."

"Goddamn it, he was just outside for a minute. I can't understand it. I was in the kitchen, getting his breakfast, when I heard all this goddamn shouting, and then gunshots, and then banging on the front door. He didn't even eat his breakfast. Has he had any? He must be starving, poor guy."

"Hercules is too sick to eat at the moment. He needs surgery as soon as possible to remove the bullet."

"Too sick to eat? That dog's never missed a meal in his life. He loves his food. Don't always have enough for me, but I always make sure that dog gets fed. He's the best damned thing that ever happened to me."

I wasn't listening. I was impatient to get out of the exam room and back to Hercules. I didn't have time for dog stories.

"Mr. Brown, we need to get Hercules to surgery. His condition is critical. I need your consent to treat him immediately."

"Surgery? I don't think Herc would like that. He's never slept a night outside his own bed. Do you think we could try something else?"

"Mr. Brown!" The old man's face gave way, a crumpling of the hope I'd seen a moment before. He gave a swift, decisive blink, and I understood the impact of my terseness.

"Mr. Brown," I said. "Our only option is surgery. If we don't get him there soon he's not going to make it."

Only minutes earlier Mr. Brown had probably been asking for directions from the bus stop to the Veterinary Hospital of the University of Pennsylvania, with no idea if Hercules was alive or dead, I realized. I'd already spent many hundreds of dollars on Hercules's care, without his owner's consent, and I was asking for permission to spend thousands more. But I wanted to save this dog, and I didn't want to let down the impatient surgeons waiting in the treatment room.

In my naïve certainty that I was doing the right thing, it didn't register that taking a bus to the hospital probably meant that Mr. Brown couldn't afford a car. That getting shot tended to happen in poorer neighborhoods. That this could be Hercules's first visit to the vet. That the cost of saving his dog's life could be more than Mr. Brown would, or could, spend on his own medical care.

I didn't tell him how much surgery and aftercare would cost. Or that his dog might die and he would be left with a several-thousand-dollar bill even if this happened.

"Do everything you can to save him," he said. He didn't pause. He didn't ask me the price of saving his dog's life. He didn't ask me the questions I'd failed to answer. I hurried from the consulting room, excited to share my success with the surgeons.


Hercules's surgery was difficult—a third of his lung was removed to control the bleeding. The small bullet hole was eclipsed by the radical median sternotomy needed to extract it—Hercules's chest was split down the middle, along his breastbone, to gain access to the injured lung. The surgery was a massive undertaking, involving a bone saw, vicious metal retractors, and surgical wire to close his chest when it was all over. I visited him in the unfamiliar ICU at the end of my shift and tried to understand the pages of treatment sheets detailing his care. I interpreted his blood gas results to see how his lungs were doing, but what I really wanted was to feel the comfort of his head in my lap.

In the first few days post-surgery, the doors of Hercules's cage stood open. This meant two things: first, he was too sick to move; and, second, there were so many fluid lines and monitoring devices attached to him that the tangle of wires and tubes made closing the doors impractical. An arterial line to monitor blood pressure snaked from his back paw. A falsely cheerful wrap in Day-Glo green around his neck hid the central line in his jugular vein, which had two different fluids hooked up to the ports. ECG pads attached to a monitor via red, black, and white wires were taped to his paws, where small rectangles of fur had been clipped to improve contact. But those were insignificant patches when compared to the huge swaths of bare skin underneath his surgical dressings.

This bewildering array ensured I kept my distance. The fierce, random alarms of the ECG machine or blood pressure monitor made me blush with guilt. I was sure that my presence, alone, had caused the noise. I was too shy to pet Hercules, afraid that I would disconnect or dislodge something essential and cause his immediate demise.

During my emergency shift I would ask Elisa tentative questions about Hercules. Her insider knowledge and friends in the ICU meant she always had the up-to-date information, but I didn't want to appear too interested. I tried to maintain a professional distance.

When I visited Hercules after my last shift of the week, the door of his ICU run was closed. His ECG leads and arterial line had been removed, and only one fluid line was connected to the venous catheter in his neck. These were all good signs—Hercules would be going home. It was likely that if he made it out of the hospital he would do well. I'd read that after a lung lobe is removed the others expand to fill the space, resulting in no long-term effects. It was improbable that the body could be so forgiving of a bullet, but watching Hercules resting comfortably in his ICU run, I could believe what the textbook said.

By my Monday shift, Hercules had been discharged. It was the first thing Elisa told me when I arrived that morning. Despite my joy that he'd made it home, a tang of sadness lingered. I wanted to know more, to have been more involved. Had his owner taken him home on the bus? Had he found a friend to give him a ride? Had Hercules licked the ICU technicians goodbye? Had Matt been the one to discharge him? I felt insignificant and excluded even though I knew that I'd fulfilled my role.

I finished my ER rotation and continued on to other departments, and when I bumped into Matt around the hospital, I would ask about Hercules. Hercules and his owner had eventually returned to have the sutures removed, a week late, Matt told me. But they didn't come back after that for follow-up visits. And the over-five-thousand-dollar bill remained unpaid.

Seeing the bullet hole in my neighbor's front door every day reminded me of Hercules. I wondered what he was doing; I hadn't known him when he was well. I didn't know the details of his life, the foods he liked, his favorite toy. I had interacted with him for a moment, yet I felt intimately connected to him.

I hadn't anticipated the emotional attachment to my patients I was experiencing, and I didn't know how to manage this aspect of being a veterinarian. There weren't any textbook chapters to explain it. It was something I was going to have to navigate on my own, along with the myriad other unexpected situations vet school hadn't prepared me for.

I'd never considered how much saving a life cost. Or how much saving a life was worth. When I was a student I'd been sheltered from the financial transactions that accompanied healthcare. In Britain, I was used to a National Health Service for human patients, and at the Royal Veterinary College most of the pet owners had purchased insurance to cover medical costs. I hadn't been aware of the economic implications of pursuing the best course of treatment. I hadn't had to think of what would happen if treatment couldn't be afforded. Now these were questions I encountered daily.

I had landed in the United States with little more than fierce determination. In the front pocket of my carry-on sat a small notebook containing what I considered to be essential veterinary information— drug dosages, differential diagnosis lists, normal blood values—which I quickly realized was useless at VHUP. I was confronted by the reality that my professional life, rather than being the scientific oasis I'd imagined, was more influenced by humanity than by medicine. The animals I had so passionately wanted to work with were only a fraction of what I was learning about. Insight into the uniquely human love for animals I'd only ever known as patients would be the most difficult, but vital, understanding I had to gain.

# CHAPTER THREE

# Monty

The handle of the cat carrier dug into my palm as we hurried along Baltimore Avenue with a lurching momentum. Monty let out an unsettling, throaty meow, and I stopped to raise the carrier and peer through the wire door at my new companion.

Monty's black, skinny body was pressed to the floor of the cage. He raised his head and stared at me with panicked ocher eyes.

"It's okay—we're almost there," I murmured and quickened my step, hustling the last few blocks. It unnerved me to be causing him such distress. I didn't have a differential list to run through, no diagnostic or treatment plan to implement. It was just my first real pet and me, making our maiden trip home.

Back at the apartment, I placed the carrier on the scuffed floor of my bedroom. The feeling of solid ground beneath Monty's feet silenced him long enough for me to realize that I, too, had been anxiously panting the whole walk home. Taking a deep breath, I made sure that the windows were closed and the bedroom door latched; I wasn't ready for Monty to meet Max and Tye, our canine roommates.

Safety checks complete, I unlocked the door of the carrier. Monty was standing at the front of the cage.

"Come on, then," I said, resisting the urge to bundle him into my arms.

A paw tentatively dabbed the floor and retracted quickly, as if testing its temperature. I waited. The same half-moon of toes padded silently onto the worn wood, followed by a leg, shoulder, and head. Carefully, the rest of his sleek body emerged. His tail flicked upward and he crouched, alert and considering his next move. The sound of German shepherd feet rushing down the corridor sent Monty scampering under the bed, leaving a trail of small moist paw prints on the floorboards.

Only a week earlier, around Halloween of my intern year, I'd received a group email sent by two veterinary students searching for a home for an older black cat they'd found wandering the streets of West Philadelphia. I'd offered to foster him for the weekend, but the name I'd chosen and the litter box, food bowl, and cat bed I'd purchased before bringing him home revealed my intentions for a more permanent relationship.

I didn't examine the implications of my decision too closely. I was several thousand miles from the place I still called home, and, for Monty, returning to England would mean a five-hour trip in the cargo hold of a plane, plus a mandatory six-month quarantine once we landed. But I had no set plans to stay in the United States beyond the year of my internship. My visa would expire in June 2001, and, only four months into my time in Philadelphia, the tang of homesickness made it difficult to imagine a future anywhere other than back across the Atlantic Ocean.

Even before I'd met Monty, I'd made space for him in my tiny bedroom and in my heart. His need for a home wasn't the only reason I responded to that email; I needed someone, or something, that would anchor me in the States; a reason to stick it out despite my loneliness. There was no shortage of social engagements to keep the hours outside the hospital filled. We had a standing Thursday night happy hour at a local sports bar. There were barbecues and parties and plastic pitchers of Yuengling or Rolling Rock after work— a uniquely American way to drink beer. But going home to my small room in the apartment I shared in name only with my intern mates kept my solitude close.

The excitement of a new country, new housemates, and new patients with new problems curdled into homesickness with the passing months of my internship. Even though I'd mastered which way to look when I crossed the street, I still hadn't found bread that tasted remotely like the sandwiches I used to eat for lunch, or the toast I'd slathered with Marmite for breakfast. I'd had no idea that one day I'd yearn for the ordinary brown bread, without high fructose corn syrup, that I'd bought on my vet student budget.

But my longing for England was in direct opposition to my furious commitment to completing my internship—and I was relying on nine pounds of black cat to tip the balance. In my mind, my determination only had to outstrip my antipathy toward wintergreen toothpaste and waxy Hershey's chocolate, the unthinkably small, essential parts of life that constantly reminded me how far I was from home.

In this sea of newness, my patients were furry islands of familiarity. American cats had the same heart rates as British ones, even though a *ginger moggy* was now an *orange domestic short-hair.* Upon abdominal palpation, their kidneys had the same firm smoothness under my nervous fingers. Their pulses had the same rapid regularity. And it was equally difficult to perform a full neurologic examination on a reluctant American or British cat.

Sometimes, however, the similarities ended in the soft nap of their coats and the warm solidity of their bodies. Diseases were different in America, especially infections carried by insects and wildlife alien to Britain, or caused by fungal agents lurking in the new ground that I walked on. I came from an island where rabies and heartworm disease didn't exist. Fungal organisms such as *Blastomyces dermatitidis* and *Histoplasma capsulatum* didn't favor British soil, and I'd never seen a case of the tick-borne Rocky Mountain spotted fever. I had to learn to recognize, diagnose, and treat these new diseases on the job, and it felt like I'd learned French from a textbook and was dumped in the middle of Paris asking for directions. I struggled to find the place for these diseases: I couldn't yet gauge their weight or texture, and I didn't know where to rank them as possible causes of my patients' illnesses.

The intake questions I'd memorized in England had to be expanded to include the administration of heartworm preventive and my patients' rabies vaccination status—first-year history-taking for the students I worked with. I vigilantly added rabies to my differential diagnosis list for any dog or cat presenting with neurologic signs such as changes in behavior, seizures, weakness, or paralysis.

One of the first decisions I faced in my new role as an owner was whether to vaccinate Monty against rabies. Despite my fears that the vaccine would cause a sarcoma—a serious tumor—at the injection site, I decided to immunize him before bringing him home. It was only one of the many unexpected choices I would run into that could affect Monty's health. I struggled with questions from whether a scented cat litter increased his risk of urinary tract problems to the best type of food for my senior, male, indoor cat. The language of animals I spoke was one of disease. I understood *normal* only in the ways it could be disrupted and altered by illness, and it was difficult to ignore my education when it came to my new pet. I saw every choice from the perspective of a veterinarian tasked with preserving life, when all I wanted was to be Monty's devoted owner. How could I expect to treat my patients if I couldn't make the right decisions for my own cat? Monty's health became another test of my veterinary skills—one I was terrified to fail.

On some level, vaccinating Monty against rabies felt superstitious, like crossing the street to avoid a black cat in my path. Rabies had always been a mythical disease to me, existing in faraway lands less fortunate than the British Isles, where it had been eradicated by 1922. It had been a hard-won battle, with tens of thousands of stray dogs slaughtered in the fight to control the disease. Such measures were not introduced for the well-being of the canine population. Rather, it was the risk to human health—the grotesque, inevitable death suffered by those bitten by a rabid dog—that demanded such aggressive control measures. Zoonoses—diseases transmitted from animals to humans—such as rabies are a side effect of living alongside animals. Whether from sharing our homes, consuming infected animal products, or encountering those carrying disease in the wild, human cases of anthrax, rabies, tuberculosis, and, in more recent times, West Nile virus and Ebola can all be traced to animal hosts.

The history of rabies and its complex role in human-canine relationships extends back millennia. In ancient Egypt, around 2000 B.C., the Laws of Eshnunna penalized with a fine of forty pieces of silver the owner of a rabid dog who bit a man. From the traditional Indian medicine of Ayurveda to Aristotle and the ancient Greeks, the terrifying specter of rabies gripped the major medical minds of progressive civilizations. Over the centuries, our fight against rabies mirrors the evolution of scientific thinking, medical practice, and our relationship with dogs.

In the 1800s, Europe was faced with a rabies epidemic. It was the height of the Industrial Revolution, and people were moving to cities such as Paris and London and bringing their dogs with them. Strays roamed the city streets, maintaining a constant viral reservoir that could easily be transmitted—by bite—to humans or their pets, with fatal consequences. Even a country's decision to slaughter stray dogs was not enough to stem the infection in mainland Europe, where rabid animals did not respect international borders.

It was Louis Pasteur, in 1885, who offered the first possibility of survival for those bitten by rabid dogs. By studying canine rabies—and accepting the personal risk that interacting with infected animals posed—he meticulously developed a vaccine that was widely administered to people and dogs. Pasteur first used the vaccine to save the life of an infected nine-year-old boy. Countless others would follow.

Heading into the twenty-first century, following the development of Pasteur's vaccine and the United Kingdom's subsequent eradication of rabies, it remained a sinister but remote threat in my home country.

In 1994, a few months before my first day at veterinary school, the Channel Tunnel connecting the United Kingdom to mainland Europe opened. Newspapers warned of an impending explosion of rabies cases when hordes of infected rats began pouring through the tunnel from France, eager to gnaw on our naïve British flesh. Wire mesh fences, electrified cattle grids, and security zones were erected to prevent the entry of adventurous, diseased animals onto British soil. But these measures did little to allay the public's concerns.

Despite the mass tabloid hysteria, the predicted epidemic did not occur. Britain remained rabies free, and the disease remained absent from my differential diagnoses lists until I saw my first patient with neurologic signs in the emergency room at VHUP.

In reality, the likelihood of encountering rabies in inner-city Philadelphia was much the same as in London. Although we were required to submit the bodies of all deceased cats and dogs with suspicious clinical signs, and those who'd died within ten days of biting a human, for mandatory rabies testing, I never encountered a case of rabies. It turned out that, although rabies was often on my differential list, it never made it to the top.

Dogs have always dominated the headlines, and the textbooks, in the discussion of rabies, with cats generally being ignored. Although cats can contract, infect others, and die from rabies, the incidence of feline-human rabies transmission has been historically insignificant. Interestingly, though, while rabies in American dogs has decreased to the point that the canine rabies variant is considered eradicated, cats accounted for 61 percent of the total number of reported rabid domesticated animals in the United States in 2014. And although feline rabies vaccination is not a legal requirement in all states, as it is for dogs, the most recent Centers for Disease Control and Prevention report recommends vaccination of all cats, dogs, and ferrets. Today, it is cats that are more likely to interact with the raccoons, skunks, and bats that still harbor the rabies virus.

Even with these numbers, there have been only thirty-four U.S. cases of human rabies since 2003, and ten of those people contracted rabies outside the United States. In developing countries with large feral dog populations, and where the cost of widespread canine vaccination programs is prohibitive, rabies remains a massively deadly disease. It is estimated that more than seventy thousand people worldwide die each year from rabies, and over 95 percent of these cases result from dog bites.

Despite my misgivings, Monty was dutifully vaccinated, examined, and blood-tested for routine health screening before I brought him home. Still, I knew I couldn't insulate him from all disease, and regardless of the choices I made for him, I couldn't prevent the inevitable. One day, he was going to get sick, with or without my veterinary degree. My understanding of disease offered no protection for my pet.

The feline medicine I'd spent years studying, however, developed a new, living dimension when I brought Monty into my life. From the pages of a textbook, or the seat of a lecture hall, disease and its consequences were abstract: something to be examined, learned, and understood. My patients were feats of biochemistry and cellular biology; I saw them on a microscopic level, a deft harmony of intricate systems borne within their skeletons. But Monty forced me to consider the dimension of disease that I'd yet to understand. His presence demanded that I acknowledge and comprehend the relationship my patients shared with the humans who brought them into my care.

From that first day, when Monty had introduced me to the particular timbre of his meow, I quickly came to look forward to the greeting he gave me each night when I got home. He would twist his long black body around my legs in tangled patterns until I sat down on the bed, so he could jump up next to me and rub his chin all over my hands in welcome. He relied on me for food, love, and a clean litter box, and I depended on him to be my family in the United States.

By the time Monty had settled in, my first patient with a gunshot wound had been superseded by a second and then a third. And bullets weren't the only projectiles I had to consider. On a later rotation through the emergency room, I'd admitted a small tortoiseshell cat, Missy, who'd been impaled by an arrow. Her owners had found her between two parked cars, missile firmly lodged from one shoulder blade to the other, cruelly resembling a character in a comedy sketch, the grubby plume of neon yellow feathers adding to the ugly absurdity of the situation.

Studying the holes in Missy's flanks where the arrow had entered and exited her body, I congratulated myself on keeping Monty as an indoor cat. Missy's thoracic cavity was almost certainly penetrated— her normal respiration a result only of the puncture wound being plugged by the arrow's shaft. Her predicament was challenging: If the arrow had passed through her chest cavity, then removal could result in instant death when air rushed in through the wound. A small crowd gathered to examine my reluctant patient, and a financial estimate was made for an emergency thoracotomy, chest tube placement, and the critical care that would follow.

This time, though, her owners shook their heads at the cost of saving their cat's life. Missy wouldn't be admitted to the ICU. I was angry over their financial limitations, and couldn't help judging their decision to let their cat outside if they couldn't afford the consequences. I wouldn't allow anything like that to happen to Monty, I told myself. The costly estimate for specialist surgery was hastily amended. We drew up a plan to remove the arrow in the emergency room, all the while praying to Bastet, Saint Gertrude of Nivelles, or whoever would listen that the arrow had missed the privileged pleural space, and passed instead through the muscle and soft tissue surrounding the spine above the chest cavity. If the gods were listening, then Missy would survive; if not, she would need immediate euthanasia.

While technicians set up for the procedure and paged the on-call surgery resident, I tried to imagine Monty on the table in front of me. I prodded at the pool of fear that washed into my stomach when I thought of Monty being injured or sick. Was that how Missy's owners felt, waiting for news of their cat? They couldn't love Missy as much as I loved Monty, I reasoned.

A brief anesthesia and a pair of bolt cutters—used to remove the tip of the arrow—allowed the surgery resident to pull the shaft straight out of Missy's body. While we held our breaths and watched her pulse oximetry reading, the numbers remained steady. Her breathing remained unchanged. She recovered fully, and the only signs of her brush with death were two small, square bald patches at the entry and exit sites. I discharged her later that day with prescriptions for pain medication and antibiotics, and my stern recommendation to keep her indoors. Despite my cool demeanor, her owners grabbed my hands in thanks, and I couldn't ignore their genuine delight and relief. Perhaps my judgment of their pet ownership had been premature.

Later that night, after my shift ended, I took up my already familiar spot sitting on the edge of the bed in my small room, waiting for Monty to join me on the mattress. He jumped onto the blanket next to me, letting out a harrumphing purr when he landed. His coat shone the brown-black of newsprint left too long in the sun.

"Good evening," I said to him. "What did you do today?"

He lay next to me and lazily stretched out a leg to place his foot on my thigh. "Really? That sounds interesting."

I lifted him onto my lap and scratched him under his bulbous chin—his favorite spot. He rubbed it vigorously against my hand, and I noticed the whiskery baldness there, like the receding hairline of an old man. I could hear a muffled game playing on the TV in the main room where I knew Chris and Dave were probably drinking beer, and the smell of cat litter reminded me that I'd forgotten to scoop Monty's box that morning. I was hungry, but I couldn't bring myself to leave the comfort of Monty and my tiny room for the vast loneliness of the TV area and kitchen. Instead I settled more comfortably on my bed, trying to not disturb Monty while I moved my leg, which was falling asleep.

I thought of Missy and wondered if she'd been kept indoors that night. "I'm never going to let you outside, ever," I said to Monty, but I realized that my promise was more to keep me safe than him. Monty had already survived an outdoor life. But his ability to jump from the floor into my arms on command wasn't a trick he'd learned on the streets. He'd clearly been someone's pet before he became mine. He'd lived a life with someone else. Someone I'd never know. Had he always been an outdoor cat and been erroneously saved by over-concerned students? Had his previous owner been an old woman who'd died alone? Did his owner get tired of him and force him out? Or did he sneak out and get lost in the unfamiliar smells of the city? I wondered if his owner had searched for him when he went missing. Did I love him more? Did he recognize the difference? Did it matter?

I caught a glimpse then, in imagining the life Monty might have led, of the empathy I'd lacked earlier in the day. The relationship my patients and their owners shared could not be measured like a blood glucose level, a white blood cell count, or the limits of a bank account. It was something less tangible, but more significant, and it was something, even with my own pet, I was only just starting to work out.


By Christmas, I'd figured out how to snatch a meager handful of time for a British reprieve from the stale monotony of Philadelphia. I'd switched shifts and begged coverage from other interns to cobble together an extra-long holiday weekend to make a trip home. I'd arranged for my roommates to take care of Monty, and I was set to travel in mid-April, just in time for Easter. I had to make it through only four months before getting the time in Hereford I'd been craving.

In my homesickness, Peter and the other veterinarians I'd seen practice with took on the shape of everything I'd left behind. The months in Philadelphia passed in a flat ubiquity of air-conditioned days inside a windowless veterinary hospital that only sharpened the bucolic memory I'd created of my hometown. It took on the essence of a Herriot book, pastoral and jolly, and my drive to leave there was forgotten in the halcyon picture I'd conjured.

The truth of my relationship with Hereford and the family I'd left behind was less shiny and peaceful. By February 2001, I'd submitted my application for an internal medicine residency, potentially committing to a further two or three years in the United States. It was a decision I'd chosen to share only once it'd been made. I was homesick, but my desire to fulfill my goals exceeded my regret about abandoning my family.

I told my mum and dad in an email that I'd applied for the U.S. residency program; that way I didn't have to hear my mum's tone, which always betrayed her emotions. I was scared to learn what she really thought, and so I didn't ask her opinion of my life-changing decision. It wasn't going to be possible to hide behind email forever, though, and the residency selection results would be out before my trip home. I would witness firsthand what my parents thought when I arrived at Heathrow. For now, though, with my future undecided, I resolved to think only about their reaction if I matched for a residency. After all, there was still a chance I'd be returning home for good in June. In the meantime, at VHUP, the routines, bureaucracy, and hierarchies had settled into my daily routine. I knew the forms for bloodwork, X-rays, and ultrasound requests, and I'd learned which members of the senior staff to avoid.

One February morning, I was on my second rotation through the internal medicine service. I sat at the nurses station waiting for the residents to arrive and assign the case transfers from the emergency room. It was a daily formality. Cases that had arrived in the ER over the preceding twenty-four hours and needed ongoing care were transferred to the appropriate service in the hospital the following morning. The residents took the bulk of the patients, to gain as much experience as possible and protect the less-experienced interns, who were spending only a month on their service.

The internal medicine department was invariably the busiest for transfers. It was the catchall for any patient with an undetermined diagnosis or plan. Animals presenting with kidney failure, liver disease, intestinal problems, or endocrine and hematologic disease were considered "regular" internal medicine transfers, but the caseload was by no means limited to patients with these conditions. There were also the unfortunate sick cats and dogs who'd been dumped in the emergency room.

Sometimes owners would bring their pets in only to disappear before a consent form or fee estimate could be signed. Other times an owner might sign paperwork and give instructions to do whatever was necessary, but subsequent phone updates would reach a disconnected number. After seventy-two hours of attempting to contact the owner, ER staff would transfer the abandoned animal to the internal medicine service for ongoing care until it was healthy enough to be sent to the city shelter, or adopted by a veterinary student, intern, or other staff member who'd grown attached while nursing it back to health.

The patient transfer sheets were instantly recognizable, printed on bright goldenrod paper, and typically arrived by 6:30 A.M. But that morning, the emergency technician hadn't brought them up to the ward yet—a crashing patient or a procrastinating, sleepy intern had delayed their arrival.

Veterinary students wearing short white coats clustered at the nurses station, or headed to the wards to check on their patients. The technicians were starting their day shifts, and the volume rose with dogs barking at their new audience and students chatting about the night before. The automatic door to the ward swung open, and ER technician Elisa strode through. She was holding the small sheaf of sheets I'd been waiting for.

"Many transfers today?" I asked.

She looked at the pages and shrugged slightly. "Not too bad for a Monday. What are you on?"

"Medicine," I replied.

"Huh. Do you like it?"

The question was loaded. She would remember my answer for my next rotation through the emergency room—her domain. The truth was that internal medicine was the place I felt most comfortable, but I wasn't about to tell her that.

"It's good," I said. "The cases are interesting. I miss the emergency room, though."

"It's pretty different up here," Elisa replied, her gaze drifting down the hall with the casual intent of a predator gauging her attack. "I'd go crazy if I was stuck doing treatments all day."

She surveyed the steady percolation of animals and people through the wards and treatment rooms. She was looking for someone. "What did you get up to this weekend?" she asked. "Any hot dates?"

"I was on pick-ups—didn't have time for anything else." I smiled, but she wasn't looking at me. I tried to guess which male student, intern, or resident was her object of interest; there weren't that many to choose from.

Elisa turned back to look at me, and I quickly dropped my eyes. "I guess you want these?" she said, flicking through the pages before handing me three sheets. She distributed the rest, a single leaf each, into the orthopedic and soft-tissue surgery boxes.

"Thanks," I said, but Elisa was already heading out of the treatment area. Relieved to finally be in possession of the transfer sheets, I turned my attention to the pages. Each sparsely typed summary contained an animal, an owner, a disease to be diagnosed, and a treatment plan to be initiated. At the top, the signalment—age, sex, breed.

At the bottom, the comments—maybe a note about financial considerations, or the last communication with the client. In between was a
brief explanation of the case, the essence of the history obtained at
two A.M. by an intern, a summary of the tests run and significant results, and the range of the financial estimate already approved. The
sheets revealed an anemic dog, a cat with a urinary tract obstruction,
and a dog with a fever of unknown origin.

Despite my developing relationship with Monty, I had yet to find
the empathy to view treating disease as something more meaningful
than the solution to a medical conundrum. Discovering the possibilities of a problem list, and the pursuit of every potential diagnosis,
was electrifying. To me, the ultimate glory lay in finding the most
obscure differential for the commonest problem.

I was intrigued by the rarest of diseases, determined to track
down every case report of conditions that had been seen in only one
or two animals. I would breathlessly suggest such diagnoses in
rounds, thrilled by the idea that I had discovered the holy grail. The
senior clinicians, however, were less impressed and would gently remind me that "when you hear hoofbeats think of horses, not zebras." It was a saying that would become etched into my memory as
a fledgling veterinarian—a useful reminder to rule out the more
common causes of a problem before reaching for the diagnostic manual. Chasing zebras rarely ended in success, and more frequently resulted in a frustrated owner left with a large bill for the diagnostic
tests performed.

Even so, I wanted to chase the esoteric. Partly because I didn't
have the experience to distinguish between common and exotic disease, but mostly because I was scared that I would miss a diagnosis by
not exploring every possibility, and in so doing cause harm to my
patient. I'd graduated vet school by studying hard, and I thought that
becoming a veterinarian required the same skills. So I tried to soothe
my anxiety by the acquisition of knowledge, and chasing zebras
worked in the same way. Although my worries weren't that easily
controlled, I continued to seek comfort in difficult internal medicine

cases. But my intern status meant that I couldn't, yet, choose the cases that I worked on, and I'd end up with the last pick after the residents.

The medicine residents were generous. They knew I wanted to join them the following year, and they'd already passed me several interesting cases. I'd experienced the addicting rush of excitement when a test confirmed a tentative diagnosis, the thrill of figuring out the relationship between lab abnormalities, clinical signs, and disease, and I was hooked. It was the cognitive challenge, the gratification of solving the puzzle, that electrified me. But I hadn't yet done my time in the isolation ward with abandoned parvo-positive puppies, or in the main medicine ward with urinary tract–obstructed cats; I had to prove myself with these cases before I could be selected for a residency.

I handed over the transfers when Mark and Tracey, the internal medicine residents, arrived at the nurses station a few minutes later. I secretly hoped for the dog with the fever of unknown origin and an extensive diagnostic workup, but I was handed the sheet for the cat, a stable patient requiring minimal testing who would probably go home in a day or two. It was the perfect case for a green intern. I glanced at the top of the paper and found my patient's name: Tiger. I wondered if he had the coat and temperament to match.

With final case transfers complete and students assigned, it was time to move our patients from the first-floor ER to the third-floor wards. Along with a better understanding of hospital hierarchy, paperwork, and how to charm the technicians, my internship had also taught me a few things about male cats with urinary tract obstructions. I was introduced to techniques and skills not covered at veterinary school: how to slide the catheter into a swollen and delicate urethra, the best sedation protocols, and the volume of intravenous fluids to give.

What I didn't know, but would come to realize, was that each hospital, and each veterinarian, had a unique way of managing these ornery patients. A specific combination of hard science and harder-to-define clinical experience wove together to form the bed of medicine on which each doctor's patients lay. After the rigidity of vet school, it was difficult to accept that experience sometimes equaled, if not surpassed, the recommended treatment regimen described in the most recent edition of *Small Animal Internal Medicine*.

I was not yet intimately acquainted with the diseases I diagnosed. I viewed them through the pages of a textbook—a table of clinical signs, typical lab abnormalities, and differential diagnoses. I made meticulous notes during rounds, while the senior clinicians discussed their preferred treatment methods, using phrases like *in my experience* and *evidence-based medicine* to justify a course of action. I spent my off-hours memorizing survival statistics from the latest *Journal of Veterinary Internal Medicine* and *Journal of the American Veterinary Medical Association*. My medicine was as definitive as the black text on the white pages of the articles I read. I understood that there was nuance, but it remained beyond my reach, buried beneath the hundreds of patients I had yet to see.

My new patient was a young cat, about three years old, who'd arrived in the emergency room the night before. His owner had rushed him in after she'd got home from work to find her healthy, energetic cat sprawled next to the litter box, barely responsive. He'd been normal that morning, if maybe a little slow to eat breakfast.

On arrival at the emergency room, Tiger's condition had prompted a stat triage. The technician answering the page would immediately have palpated his abdomen to assess his urinary bladder. Running her hands from behind his rib cage toward his tail, she would've encountered the turgid tennis ball of his dangerously enlarged bladder; he'd been struggling to urinate for hours, a gritty plug of cells, protein, and crystals obstructing his urethra.

The technician's announcement of "He's blocked!" triggered a well-established routine: crash cart, IV catheter and fluids, blood gas measurement, sterile gloves, lube, tiny Tomcat urinary catheter, sterile saline for flushing all set up within a few minutes. His heart rate had been precariously low, his heart muscle cells stuporous from the massive amount of potassium circulating in his blood. Toxins and metabolic by-products that should've been excreted hours before were accumulating in a poisonous stew. I pictured Tiger lying in the emergency room, ECG hooked up, intravenous fluids and drugs to stabilize his heart running through a line into his vein, a technician shouting out the blood results that flashed up on the screen. I was relieved that it hadn't been my shaky hands placing the urinary catheter. Tiger had stabilized overnight, his blood potassium, urea nitrogen, and creatinine slowly returning to normal with the large volumes of intravenous fluids he received.

My job over the next few days was to keep watch over Tiger, continue to flush the toxins out of his body, and, at the critical moment, pull the urinary catheter and ensure he could urinate on his own. Timing was crucial. Remove the catheter too soon and re-blockage could occur, necessitating more time in the hospital and the possible euthanasia of a young cat with owners unprepared for such expense.

Over the past few months, my thoughts, increasingly, had turned to Monty when considering my patients. I knew he spent most of his day asleep, safely sequestered in my small bedroom. He probably woke for the occasional snack of dry food, or to use the litter box I'd positioned in the farthest corner from my bed. Was that how Tiger had been spending his days? For Tiger, a sedentary, indoor lifestyle and dry food diet had caused him to get a little plump around the middle. I thought of Monty's growing belly. This, along with Tiger's gender and genetics, had likely caused the blockage that had endangered his life. Neutered male, indoor, overweight cats, eating dry food, and peeing in a box were the typical patients to develop feline lower urinary tract disease, which could culminate in the life-threatening urethral obstruction that had brought Tiger to VHUP.

I doubted Tiger's owner had considered any of these factors when she'd decided to own a cat. I, on the other hand, at times could think of nothing else. Should Monty be an outdoor cat if that decreased his chances of developing a urethral obstruction? Should I feed him inconvenient, smelly canned food instead of the kibble I shook into his bowl every day?

I'd decided that Monty wasn't going to be an outdoor cat, but the dry food I rattled into his bowl every morning spiked a more intense ambivalence. For some cats wet food was better, but the inconvenience of can openers and half-finished cans in the refrigerator was unappealing, as was the expense on an intern's salary. I was a veterinarian, and my choices as a pet owner potentially put my cat at an increased risk of developing urinary tract problems because dry food was cheaper and more convenient. Practicing perfect cat husbandry had seemed easy sitting in a lecture hall, but Monty was teaching me that it wasn't so simple.

I identified Tiger by the empty bag outside his ER cage slowly filling with fluid. Were it not for the attachment to the urinary catheter, I wouldn't have recognized it as urine. It was strawberry-hued, and small islands of blood clots and cellular debris turned the bag into a macabre snow globe. *That's one pissed-off bladder,* I thought, crouching in front of the cat. My patient's horizontal ears and immediate growl told me it wasn't just his bladder that was pissed off.

Tiger was flattened against the back of his cage. He didn't take his eyes off me. I reached for his treatment sheet, and his rumbling growl peaked into an indignant hiss. His pupils were so dilated from adrenaline that I couldn't discern the color of his eyes. He was a gray-brown tabby, with the tigerish stripes his name foretold. The white Elizabethan collar he wore to prevent him from removing his catheters lent a vaguely comedic cast to his rage. His face, framed by the plastic moon, reminded me of a sulking child in a school play. His black plume of a tail was deflated and bedraggled, but the tip flicked a warning that echoed his growl.

Treatment sheet in hand, I stepped back from the cage. Reviewing his fluid shifts over the past twelve hours, I looked over his urine output, tallied his fluid input, and calculated the difference, acutely aware that I was delaying the moment of opening his cage door.

The temperament of my patients was a bewildering addition to my problem list, a confounding factor that rarely worked in my favor. Frightened cats and dogs could be aggressive or stupefied, influencing the findings on physical examination and preventing the discovery of potentially vital clues. Despite Tiger and Monty's similarities, they seemed separated by more than the few blocks it took to walk to the hospital each morning. Tiger's fear, discomfort, and trip to the emergency room had changed him into a feral animal.

Over-exuberant, friendly pets could prove equally challenging. A young, energetic chocolate Labrador retriever had taught me earlier that year that temperament wasn't always a good assessment of disease severity. He'd greeted me with a vigorous lick and tail wag, and then dragged me, on the end of his leash, down the corridor to radiology, where an ultrasound confirmed an overwhelming, life-threatening infection in his abdominal cavity due to a barbeque skewer piercing his intestine. He'd skipped breakfast that morning—a never-before-witnessed event—then vomited and seemed out of sorts, but the excitement of a car ride to the hospital had overridden his discomfort. Fortunately, his insuppressible energy meant that he was discharged the day after surgery with no complications.

I proceeded cautiously with Tiger. How could I perform a physical examination on a patient growling so loudly that I couldn't hear his heart or lung sounds? How could I interpret a cat's behavior when he was too frightened to do anything other than huddle in the corner of his carrier?

When I was a student I'd been protected—there'd always been a more senior veterinarian or technician to intervene if the patient became too difficult. Now, I was responsible not only for the safety and well-being of Tiger, but also of the staff and students he interacted with.

"Monty would never act like this," I muttered, looking warily at Tiger.

I considered my options for getting us both safely to the third-floor ward. Large towel? Cat gloves? Muzzle? This wasn't the first time I'd felt inadequate in front of a twelve-pound patient. Asking for help seemed like admitting defeat, but I also didn't want to get bitten. I felt an irrational flame of rage at Tiger's low growl, fueled by my awareness of the damage he could inflict if I didn't handle the situation appropriately. I wondered if his rabies vaccination was up to date.

Time was running out. I'd been in the emergency room for fifteen minutes, and Tiger was no closer to transfer. Other patients and their coteries of students, interns, and residents had already left. My assigned student was missing, either busy with ward duties or loitering in a hallway having caught wind of our patient's temper. Regardless, this was my responsibility. The buck—or tomcat—stopped with me.

I tried summoning calm, hoping to dispel the tension with wishful thinking. I imagined what George would do—the lilt of his Scottish burr quietly reassuring his frightened patient. The capable breadth of his hands dwarfing even the largest and angriest cats.

But summoning old mentors and wishful thinking weren't going to alter my patient's mood, or magic him upstairs and into the internal medicine ward. Instead, I had to rely on the help at hand; I needed to call on Elisa. I scanned the emergency room for any other technicians, but my attempt was halfhearted. Elisa was experienced and, when it came to handling an aggressive cat, I knew she could get Tiger out of his cage without significant damage to him or to us. I wrestled my pride down far enough to allow a deference to Elisa to rise before I walked toward her. Her ready response to my request suggested that she'd known I was going to need her help, but I hung on to my smile and listened to her expound on the best ways to handle a cross cat.

With the swift dexterity of an experienced cat wrangler, Elisa pinned Tiger to the back of his cage with a large, dense blanket. The thick fabric shielded us from claws and teeth and muffled his escalating wail. In one quick movement she swept the blanket between him and the cage wall so he was wrapped completely in the material—an unpleasant burrito. She placed my very displeased patient on the waiting gurney, holding him in the blanket while I hastily grabbed his fluid pump and urinary catheter bag, trying to avoid yanking on any of his lines and causing a crisis. Once we started our unceremonious procession to the third floor ward, Tiger's anger had abated, likely overcome by confusion at this new adventure.

Throughout his stay Tiger was a challenging patient. He tested my confidence when his fierce demeanor forced me to concede my inability to perform a physical examination every morning. He tested my nerve when he chewed out and swallowed his urinary catheter the morning it was due to be removed. I administered an emetic and waited fifteen nerve-racking minutes for it to take effect. I'd never been so happy to see a patient vomit.

At discharge, he was so difficult to take out of his cage that I asked his owner to come up to the wards to coax him into his carrier. I hovered a few feet away from Tiger's cage while his owner—an ordinary middle-aged woman—approached. She was quiet and seemed nervous in the hospital, and I feared she was no match for Tiger's ferocity. If he bit her, I would be responsible. She knelt in front of his cage and placed the carrier on the floor beside her. For a moment Tiger didn't move, and then he noticed her and approached the front of the cage, flicking his tail in the air and rubbing his face and the length of his body along the cage door.

"Tiger," she said. "My handsome boy, I've been so worried about you."

He chirruped a meow at her voice. She opened the cage door and he dropped his head into her open hand.

"You ready to go home?" she asked. And when she opened the carrier he hopped in.

Something tight and unfamiliar caught in my chest when I watched Tiger with his owner. The animal I'd felt at war with, the medical problem I'd tried to solve, was suddenly a different creature. He was more than an angry bundle of fur with a urinary catheter; he was loved. I hadn't possessed the right lens to see the essential, emotional connection each of my patients shared with their owners until

Monty arrived. And I was still figuring out how to incorporate this new information into my practice. But the weight of Monty on my bed at night, the vital warmth of him in my arms and the discovery of the need I felt for him, demanded that I see the animals I cared for in a different way.

# CHAPTER FOUR

# Fritz

O n Match Day in mid-March 2001, I learned I would be staying at the University of Pennsylvania for at least two more years. The Veterinarian Internship and Residency Matching Program, or "the Match," was the official program all intern and resident candidates applied to for a position at their preferred institutions. Through a combination of candidate and hospital rankings and a complex, mystical algorithm, positions were assigned in a method that seemed effective, but always provided enough confusing outcomes to obscure exactly how the system worked. Luckily, I had ranked Penn as my first choice, and I was excitedly relieved to be starting my internal medicine residency there in June.

Philadelphia was finally becoming my home, and I wasn't ready to trade it for another locale. It was not as unlike a British city as I'd first perceived. I'd found a tiny bakery next to a small park, Rittenhouse Square, that made the most delicious bread. I could walk there on a weekend day, and it reminded me of my time in central London.

I'd settled on my favorite breakfast place, which was tucked into a beautiful Victorian home in the gritty center of West Philadelphia, and my friends had introduced me to the trails in Fairmount Park— a hidden oasis on the banks of the Schuylkill River with areas so densely wooded you couldn't hear the traffic on the nearby freeway. On a good day, I could forget I wasn't in England. My belongings had expanded beyond the two suitcases I'd checked on my flight from London, and my loneliness had been allayed by Monty's arrival.

Most of the interns in my class had applied for residencies— surgery, cardiology, internal medicine, oncology, critical care. The choice of specialty varied, but the significance of residency Match Day was the same. It was a day of absolutes: elation or despondency; acceptance or rejection. Those who were chosen had the next few years mapped out. But for the one or two who were passed over, plans had to be remade, goals flattened, and disappointments swallowed.

Regardless of the social strata of my intern class, which had solidified over the months of our internship, Match Day was an accepted moment of obligated camaraderie. After clinics that day, we met at a Mexican restaurant a few blocks from the hospital for a dangerous mix of margaritas, commiseration, and celebration. Between the second and third round of drinks the muted delight of those who'd been matched and the fake cheer of those who hadn't began to dissolve like the salt rims on our glasses. The group divided, with the couple of interns who hadn't applied attempting to bridge the gap. But by the fourth round, a diffuse melancholy had settled on our group as we mulled the nine months we'd spent together, and considered the years that lay ahead.

I felt a part of something that night. I stood on shared ground with my fellow interns; I understood their disappointment and joined their celebration. We'd come from different places, and after sharing a year of saving and ending lives, pushing the boundaries of our knowledge, skill, and emotional resilience, we were headed to different futures.

My long-expected trip home in April acquired a particular significance when I found out I'd be staying in the United States for my
residency. Over the next two years, this would be how I saw England
and my family—in sporadic gulps of time snatched and cobbled together via short trips across the Atlantic. My preoccupation with the
residency match and the long days on clinics meant that I'd had little
time to consider that the place I was going home to may have changed
from the one I'd left behind.

In the early months of 2001, a crisis was unraveling in the United
Kingdom—one that would forever change the fabric of my hometown and the British veterinary profession I'd known. The first case
of foot and mouth disease (FMD) in Britain since 1967 was diagnosed
on February 19, 2001. Like rabies, it was a scary but distant vet school
disease. We'd learned about it with somber and dire warnings, but
had never expected to see or diagnose a case. The consequences of
FMD, though, are more complex than the inevitable death awaiting
those infected with rabies. FMD is a large-animal disease—exclusively
affecting cloven-hooved livestock such as cattle, sheep, and pigs—and
the virus, which is airborne, is easily and rapidly transmitted, like the
common cold. The disease is rarely fatal, and those infected can fully
recover; however, it causes weight loss and decreased milk production due to painful, debilitating oral and pedal ulcers.

For decades prior to the outbreak, the United Kingdom had been
free of the disease without preventive vaccination. This gave the
country a privileged position in the export of livestock, with a significant financial advantage. The 1980 European Union regulations pro-
hibited the export of any animals exposed to the virus due to the
severe economic consequences of an infection. EU countries with
endemic disease could vaccinate their livestock to prevent infection
until 1992, when the European Union banned the use of the vaccine
because testing could not distinguish vaccinated from infected animals. This meant that when the disease was detected in the United

Kingdom in 2001, the method for controlling the virus was to kill all infected and possibly exposed livestock. It was a purely economic decision, to protect the United Kingdom's disease-free status, made with little regard for the welfare of the livestock involved, or the farmers who cared for them.

By the time the first case was diagnosed the disease had already spread from the farm it was initially detected on—through the transport of infected pigs—across the countryside. When I heard the news a few days later, FMD had traveled from northern England to Herefordshire, more than two hundred miles away. I thought of the many farms I'd visited with Peter. I thought of my high school friend whose family owned a dairy and sheep farm on the Welsh border—the place I'd learned to dehorn calves, milk cows, and skid around a paddock at night searching for lambing ewes by the headlights of the pickup we rode in.

Between the news of the first case in February and my April trip to the United Kingdom, I wondered what I would've done if I'd stayed in England. Would I have volunteered to inspect animals for signs of disease? Would I be signing the slaughter notices of those infected? Enforcing the cull of all livestock within the three-kilometer contiguous zone around the affected farm?

After I met my dad at the airport, being in England felt like I was taking a deep breath after puffing through a straw for ten months. I recognized the voice of the DJ on Radio One; we were driving on the right—the *correct*—side of the road, and at the motorway services I stocked up on bottles of Ribena, bags of Walkers salt and vinegar crisps, and any kind of chocolate other than Hershey's. We chatted about the family events I'd missed—my grandma's eightieth birthday party, my sister's new teaching job in Bournemouth—and a lightly polished version of my life in Philadelphia. When we left the urban sprawl of London and headed west to Hereford, I became aware of an insidious stillness hovering over the passing countryside. When I looked across the fields, it seemed that the skyline had been rubbed out with a dirty eraser, the distinction between land and sky hazy and gray.

The dairy and beef cattle, ewes and month-old lambs that had been as much part of the landscape as the fields and hedgerows had vanished. Since seeing practice with Peter, I'd sewn the livestock deeply into the fabric of the land. My experience had reshaped the anonymous herds into a network of farmers, herdsmen, milking parlors, and lambing sheds. The empty fields symbolized more than the absence of their usual inhabitants. Each represented a fragment of a shattered community, a decimated livelihood.

At the height of the FMD crisis, 80,000 to 93,000 animals were slaughtered weekly in an effort to control viral spread. But the government's efforts to contain the virus unwittingly contributed to the persistence of the disease across the land. Infected carcasses were driven through uninfected areas, causing spread of the pathogen, and it was ultimately discovered that aerosolization of the virus during cremation resulted in dissemination, rather than destruction, of the viral particles.

From the car window, as we traveled closer to Hereford, I noticed that the haze I'd seen earlier had transformed into a denser, black smoke. I clung to the possibility that farmers were burning stubble on arable land, or incinerating waste, but the acrid, terrible smell of burning hair, fleece, and hooves that seeped through the car's air vents betrayed the smoke's true origin. The infrastructure to dispose of the vast number of dead animals didn't exist, and makeshift pyres smoldered across the landscape, bodies burning upon the land they'd once grazed.

It was hard to grasp the devastation. These were small family-run farms, passed down through generations—100 to 150 cows, and perhaps a couple of hundred sheep. I'd met these farmers and witnessed how intimately they knew their animals; their dairy cows had names, personalities, and idiosyncrasies. They could predict the particular order their herd would walk into the milking shed, and remembered where each cow most liked to be scratched.

I realized, driving home that day, and again during my stay in Hereford—the weekly cattle market canceled, all country walking trails closed—that British farming and my home would forever be changed by the FMD crisis. The impact stretched far beyond the farm gates: Country pubs and village shops were shuttered; the fear of viral transmission on clothing and footwear had paralyzed the rural economy.

And then there was the human cost: the sixty suicides, the epidemic of depression that hit the farming community, and the loss of more than 7,800 jobs. The damage to the British economy was priced at £8 billion, split between the private and public sectors, a figure that included loss of tourism due to the closure of the countryside. Six million animals were slaughtered, but it was six months before the last case was diagnosed, on September 30, 2001, and almost twelve months before the final sheep were killed in January 2002.

The distance created by the nine months I'd spent in the United States stopped me from reaching out to Peter and the farmers I'd met. My clinical life in Philadelphia was intensely focused on monitoring tenths of a point change in lab parameters, while livestock in the United Kingdom were being slaughtered by the thousands, on the farms where the farmers lived, and would go on living, even after their animals were gone. My idyllic, homesick imaginings fractured from the terrible truth of a crisis I was not a part of, and an experience from which I was isolated.

I had been changed by my move to the United States, and my leaving had changed what I considered home. I couldn't hold on to my memories of England; the country they represented no longer existed.

After I'd slept off some of my jet lag and drunk enough English beer to remind myself of how a real pint should taste, it was time for my return trip to Heathrow. I'd missed Monty when I'd slept in my childhood bed every night, but going back to the States was hard. To ease my return to Philadelphia, I'd stocked my suitcase with minty toothpaste, Marmite, Wotsits, and English chocolate. I waved good-bye to my dad at the airport gate with promises to phone more, email more, and take care of myself. We didn't talk about when I would visit again; neither of us acknowledged that my future—whatever it would be—was waiting for me across the ocean.

Monty was happy to see me when I arrived back in Philadelphia, and his presence was a greater comfort than I'd anticipated. The last weeks of my internship passed in a similar flurry to those that had preceded it, and over one weekend in mid-June 2001 I graduated from intern to resident. My internal medicine residency began with a lecture about responsibility, commitment, privilege, and expectation by the director of VHUP. I paid cursory attention to his rousing words, instead trying to calm the nauseous trepidation that fizzed in my stomach and identify my fellow internal medicine residents among the other white coats. I was preparing for battle with my contemporaries, but if I'd stepped back I would've realized that the only competitor was me. The satisfaction of obtaining exactly what I wanted was undermined by my unrelenting desire for personal perfection, and the certainty that I couldn't achieve it.

Monty and I moved into a one-bedroom with a bathroom and kitchen all to ourselves, financed by my barely increased resident salary. The new place was a few blocks away from the hospital, and it was a relief to be out of the old one. I'd never bonded with my roommates, and even at the hospital the distance between us grew. Following our internship, Chris escaped the confines of academia to work in a private emergency practice in the Pacific Northwest, and, though Dave was staying for a surgery residency at Penn, there was never the assumption that we would continue to share our living space.

The apartment was on the seventh floor of what, from a distance, looked like a stately older building. The mellow brick, the uniform rows of windows with pale stone accents, and the large gated court-yard that led to the impressive main entrance lent the place grandeur. Up close, however, the window frames were chipped and yellowed. The pieces of cardboard, old towels, and various items of clothing that were stuffed around air conditioners occupying every other window told a more accurate story.

The building was popular accommodation for graduate students, interns, and residents, and I had lucked into a corner unit through a friend of a friend. Monty had a window to sit in, birds to watch, and swaths of sunlit floor to recline on. His litter box was now more than a foot from my bed, and we enjoyed breakfast together in the small dining area off the galley kitchen. It was the first time I'd lived in my own apartment and, although the cupboards didn't close completely and a generation of dust occupied the space under the stove, I felt lucky. I'd chosen the shower curtain and bath mat, and arranged my toiletries on the slim window ledge behind the sink. The fridge con-tained only my food. My new apartment had been furnished through the kindness of final-year residents who were moving on; I got a free couch, coffee table, dining table, and chairs to fill what would other-wise have been an empty space.

Monty still slept on the end of my bed, creating a permanent warm, hairy divot in the blanket. I continued to worry about his health. I urgently scheduled bloodwork and an abdominal ultrasound when he lost weight, only to realize that his new look was a result of the diet food I had accidentally purchased.

I had an apartment and a competitive small-animal internal medi-cine residency. I had a ready-formed cadre of friends, and within that group I found those with whom I'd share dinners and drinks, and celebrate Thanksgiving and Christmas, and to whom I'd go to for advice on tough cases. But, despite this, at times I felt terrifyingly alone.

Under the carapace of bright, eager energy I showed the world, I was at war. I snapped at the inexperienced vet students and testily disagreed with my fellow residents during rounds in an effort to prove myself. Then I spent evenings fretting over every time I'd cracked.

Now that I'd achieved resident status, each new patient felt like a final exam to be failed. They were problems to be investigated in exhaustive lists. They were diagnoses to be nailed, treatment plans to be initiated, and discharges to be written. They were opportunities to gain the approval of senior clinicians and fellow residents that I relentlessly sought at case rounds.

Transitioning from vet school to internship to residency was like learning to ride a bike only to discover that what was required was to unicycle backward, while wearing a blindfold and juggling. In every facet, becoming a resident demanded more than I'd thought possible. It wasn't only the challenges of increased case responsibility, greater diagnostic independence, and higher expectations for clinical excellence that separated my first and second years at Penn.

The rotating structure of the internship had shielded me from long-term case management and the development of deeper client relationships, which were the foundation my internal medicine career would be built on. Now there would be no moving on after a month, no ducking out of a difficult case, no citing inexperience. And the emotional stakes were higher than I'd foreseen; my patients were loved family pets, sole companions, and child substitutes that I became desperate to save for their people. They had finally become singular creatures beyond the diseases they carried, making my role as their doctor vital on a complex new level.

A few months into my residency I'd established a daily routine, which was often interrupted by the beep of my pager signaling the constant demands of the sick animals under my care. My schedule was dictated by those goldenrod transfer sheets, which foretold the number and types of cases that would occupy each day. I still felt an undeniable excitement each transfer morning, a frisson of delight with each sheet and the internal medicine problems that were hidden between the lines.

One morning I picked up a sick young dog. On presentation to the emergency room—a little less than twenty-four hours before his transfer into my care—Fritz was just another dog who'd eaten something he shouldn't have. Countless canines arrived at the hospital after gobbling socks and wallets, cassette tapes, balls and other toys, unopened ten-pound bags of dog, cat, and even bird food, and disgusting rotten trash can contents best left unidentified. Not to mention those dogs who came in because of something their owners had fed them, often confessed only on the third round of questioning:

"Are you sure he couldn't have got into anything?"

"Well, there was that Wendy's hamburger, fries, and shake I shared with him on Friday, but that wouldn't make him sick, would it?"

The answer was always "Yes."

The morning Fritz arrived he hadn't been interested in breakfast, a peculiarity rare enough to raise an alarm for his owner. When he'd started vomiting she'd rushed him to the emergency room. Factoring in "dog years," Fritz, at three, and his owner, who was a young graduate student, were about the same age and were constant companions. He was a black and tan miniature dachshund. The sharpness of his pointed nose was softened by his overlarge, floppy ears and his dark, fluid eyes. He had the tight glossy coat of a well-cared-for pet.

The intern who'd examined Fritz noted that he was quiet and dehydrated, with discomfort on abdominal palpation. On closer history-taking, it emerged that Fritz and his owner, who shared most things, had shared a hot dog a day or so before the trouble began.

There wasn't an algorithm that could predict the outcome for dogs with "dietary indiscretion." Breed, body weight, matter ingested, or frequency of ingestion didn't appear to influence the probability of life-threatening complications. A poor pulse, high heart rate, and fever could indicate that further steps were needed—X-rays to look for an intestinal obstruction, bloodwork for signs of infection, or abdominal ultrasound to interrogate the abdominal organs. More often than not, though, the signs were vague. A patient's elevated heart rate might be due to the car ride to the hospital and the scent of hundreds of other pets who'd passed through the emergency room. A faint pulse could be the result of nothing more than a timid intern's fingers, but it could also mean that dehydration or shock was causing low blood pressure. Or it could be just another dog with garbage gut who'd been getting into the trash again, with no more serious repercussions than vomit on the carpet.

Fritz's discomfort and signs of nausea—lip licking and smacking, as though he had a bad taste in his mouth—recommended his admission to the hospital. His owner had readily agreed, with the confidence of a student who was used to her parents picking up the tab. A strip of fur on Fritz's leg was clipped for intravenous catheter placement, and his treatments of intravenous fluids, antibiotics, and medications to control his pain and nausea were started. The results of his bloodwork showed dehydration and an elevated white cell count— a sign of possible inflammation or infection—but there was no evidence of an intestinal obstruction on his X-rays. These results illuminated what Fritz couldn't tell us: He was sick, and the decision to admit him to the hospital was the right one.

When I met Fritz for the first time he looked depressed—quiet, uninterested, and with low energy. He'd continued to vomit overnight and he had the queasy look of a reluctant sailor. He lay on his side, facing the back of his cage, and his only reaction to my approach was a disinterested flick of his ear. When I gently slid my hands under his slim body to pick him up, I felt a tense tremor that told me he was in pain. His back was instinctively arched to protect his abdomen, and a sticky gum of saliva coated his chin, reflecting his persistent nausea. His pulse was rapid—he wasn't depressed from being away from home overnight; his elevated heart rate told me that his body was at battle. The soft skin of his abdomen felt too warm, and his last body temperature had been above the normal range—another sign he was deteriorating despite treatment.

I was learning to rely on my clinical skills—the information I could acquire with my hands, ears, and eyes by listening to a heart, interpreting a patient's demeanor, and palpating an abdomen—in the same way that I'd relied on the diagnoses I'd memorized. I was gaining a wary trust of my gut feeling when something didn't look right, and I was worried about Fritz.

My biggest concern, having taken Fritz's physical examination, bloodwork, and X-rays into consideration, was that he had a condition called pancreatitis, an inflammation of the pancreas.

The pancreas is a complex organ, nestled between the duodenum— part of the small intestine—and stomach. It is intimately associated with the bile duct and lies close to the gallbladder and liver. Early in my training, when I still spent time in surgery suites, the mantra for abdominal exploratories was always *Don't piss off the pancreas*. Like an irritable aunt at Christmas dinner, the merest look or touch could set off an angry inflammation. To me, the pancreas appeared pale and malevolent, hiding between the smooth, jolly pink intestines and the dense, bloody liver, a lumpy narrow irregularity of tissue waiting to catch an inexperienced surgeon out. An organ with its temperament doesn't belong in the busy abdominal cavity; its pallid friability would be better suited to a more protected space. But there it is, secreting insulin and other hormones into the bloodstream and digestive enzymes into the gut.

In patients with pancreatitis, the meticulous delivery of enzymes to the intestine is disrupted by inflammation, which can be triggered by genetics, something indiscernible, or even a fatty meal, including a hot dog, fried chicken, or Bloomin' Onion snatched from a kitchen counter, dug out of a trash can, or offered as a reward. In humans, the most common trigger of pancreatitis is alcohol consumption. This inflammation sends enzymes designed to digest food into the pancreas itself, the surrounding tissue, and, if things get bad, into the bloodstream. Enzymes do not discriminate, and once they escape their carefully marshaled delivery to the intestine they digest the pro-teins and fats wherever they land, a potentially catastrophic event that has little effective treatment.

I knew Fritz's pancreatitis could confound every medical interven-tion I mustered against it and, although I could explain, pathophysi-ologically, every inflammatory pathway and its consequences, I knew that I might not be able to save him.

After I settled Fritz in the wards, persuaded the radiology techni-cian to bump his ultrasound to the top of the list, and warned my student to contact me if Fritz's condition changed, I headed to my office to call his owner. The internal medicine residents' office was at least twice the size of the broom closet the interns shared. Each of the eight residents had a cubicle with a desk, computer, and phone. I decorated my cube with animal-themed newspaper cartoons clipped from The Guardian by my parents, and pictures and cards sent by the owners of my current and former patients—each one a small paper trophy affirming my worth.

Despite the solace I found in the cards, they carried their own sad-ness. The deepest thanks came from the owners of those I wasn't able to save—animals who had been too sick to be helped, whom I'd euthanized, or who'd died despite my intervention. Sometimes I'd open a card and find a glossy photograph of my patient from happier times, healthy and vibrant, as their owner had known them. A calico cat sitting in her favorite sun spot, a black cocker spaniel dressed like a devil for a Halloween parade. Markers of a time in a pet's life when veterinarians and hospitals were far away.

Regardless of the relative luxury of my new office space, making calls to owners was my least favorite part of the day. I felt a confusing ambivalence toward the humans in my patients' lives, and I struggled to figure out how they fit into my practice. Their financial constraints limited the tests I could run and the treatments I could administer. And, even when money was no object, I felt inadequate to meet their expectations. People had emotional needs I didn't understand and couldn't navigate, and they required my time and patience, which I didn't have enough of.

My veterinary school education hadn't encompassed bedside manner, or owner communication skills. Humans had barely figured in our lectures—pet owners were anonymous beings who brought Fluffy and Fido to the hospital when something wasn't right, and picked them up again when everything was better. Case studies were presented with a picture of the animal patient alone, in a vacuum, without human interference or companionship.

The expertise needed to counsel a grieving client, find the right words to explain a complicated disease to a layperson, or understand that an owner's anger was often a manifestation of fear, were not re-quirements for graduation. To become a board-certified internal medicine specialist, I had to complete a residency, author a journal article, write three case reports, and pass two written examinations. There were procedures to master, diseases to diagnose and conquer, and standards of care to attain. These were measurable parameters, specific criteria to be fulfilled before the letters *DACVIM* (Diplomate of the American College of Veterinary Internal Medicine) could be tacked to the end of my name. Even through this advanced stage of training, owner communication remained little more than an ab-stract, a mysterious art absent from any training manual or rounds discussion.

The language we spoke in case rounds, in the wards to discuss patients, and in the basement lecture theater for grand rounds, was comforting in its precision. The Latin derivations made diseases that were ugly and sad seem exotic. Devastating, life-ending complica-tions hid behind benign-sounding acronyms like DIC—disseminated intravascular coagulation, or, more realistically, *death is coming.* The visceral reality of watching a patient die from uncontrollable hemor-rhage, or witnessing the suffocating distress of severe pulmonary edema, was lost in the formality of our academic language.

During my residency, I was discovering that this vocabulary was meaningless in the exam room. Using complex medical terminology resulted only in an owner's confusion, and often a loss of their consent. I had to be an interpreter—both of what my client could and couldn't tell me, and of what the test results and diagnoses meant to an owner who was terrified for the future of their pet. I had to find a common language for the sake of my patient, who couldn't speak, and doing that was harder than any exam I'd taken.

Fritz's owner answered my call on the first ring. I suspected that she'd been waiting by the phone.

"Good morning. This is Dr. Suzy Fincham calling from the Veterinary Hospital of the University of Pennsylvania. I'm Fritz's new—"

"How is he?" The voice on the other end of the line was high-pitched and panicked.

"He's stable, but I'm a little worried about his condition," I replied.

"Why? What happened?"

My grip on the receiver tightened. I paused, immediately ruffled by the accusation I heard in her question.

"Ms. Whitney," I continued, "nothing has happened to Fritz. He's been transferred to the internal medicine service, and I'm his new doctor."

"But, how is he?" *You're demanding,* I thought. "Can I come and visit?"

I switched the receiver to my other ear and pushed my weight back in my chair. I wanted to discuss Fritz as a patient. I wanted to review his medical history and lay out my treatment and diagnostic recommendations in the clinical terms I felt most comfortable speaking, but his owner needed something else from me.

"He's going to be okay, isn't he?" she continued. "You can fix him, right? He's my baby. You won't let anything bad happen to him, will you?"

"I think Fritz has pancreatitis," I replied. "We will do an ultrasound of his abdomen today to confirm this, but at the moment this is what we're treating him for."

"What? Pancreitis? I thought he just had an upset stomach. He was fine two days ago. Is he going to die?"

I felt the pull of her anxiety dragging the conversation away from the medical territory I was trying to maintain. "Pancreatitis can be serious, and in some cases life-threatening, but—"

"He seemed fine when I left yesterday. Now you're saying he's going to die?"

I swallowed, hearing panic rising in her voice.

"No, no, Ms. Whitney, I didn't say Fritz is going to die. I just said that he has a potentially serious disease."

She began sobbing, and my voice trailed off. I didn't know how our conversation had gone so quickly from "hello" to Fritz's death, and I was equally unsure of how to pull it back to a place of calm. I wanted to hang up and transfer Fritz's care to one of the other residents, sure that they would be able to establish a relationship where I had failed.

I could intently monitor Fritz's clinical progress over the next twenty-four hours. I could adjust his medications to control his pain and nausea. I could sit with him and feel the smooth softness of his ears. I could care for my patient, but I didn't know how to do the same for his owner.

"An abdominal ultrasound will allow us to get a good look at his pancreas and the rest of his organs," I continued. "We will also monitor his white blood cell count and liver enzymes, and we will increase his medications, because he still seems uncomfortable and nauseous. Once I've got more information, I'll give you a call and then we can set up a visit. Does that sound okay?"

"Yes," came her hiccupped reply.

"The business office will call you with an updated estimate, and I'll speak to you later."

"It doesn't matter what it costs. Do whatever it takes to save him."

"Try not to worry" was the only reply I could muster. As I hung up, my pager went off, informing me that Fritz was headed to ultrasound, stat.

In case rounds later that day we discussed pancreatitis. We debated the benefits of fresh frozen plasma and intravenous nutrition. We reviewed journal articles and scientific papers, paying attention to mortality rates, predictors of survival, and potential new treatments. I tried to focus on the discussion, but my mind kept drifting to Fritz, in cage 7. I thought of how he'd made small, uncomfortable grunts with each exhale during his ultrasound. How he'd developed leaking, greenish-black diarrhea. How he continued to vomit despite the multiple anti-emetics he was receiving. I didn't like how he was doing, and I didn't like the prospect of discussing this with his distressed owner.

At the end of rounds, I lingered to ask my senior clinician his advice. Dr. Goldman was a full professor and a world leader in veterinary gastroenterology. He was a short, compressed man. Dark hair cut close to his head, tight full beard—even his glasses seemed to absorb into his face rather than adorn it. His clothes were cut economically; nothing was extraneous.

"Dr. Goldman? I was wondering if I could get your opinion on something?"

He was already halfway to his office, and once the door was closed I wouldn't have the nerve to bother him, but I was hoping he might share some wisdom to improve my relationship with Fritz's owner.

"Dr. Fincham, very interesting case you've got there, nasty bit of pancreatitis. What was it he ate? A hamburger?"

"A hot dog. His owner thought it was a treat. She's very worried about him."

"I'm sure you've reassured her with your plan," he replied. "She's right to be worried about her little dog. I'm heading to the lab to check on some experiments, but then I'll be in the wards. Come and find me if you have any other questions."

"Thank you," I managed to force out before watching him stride away. I was eager to make a good impression, and I didn't have the courage to prolong our conversation. Dr. Goldman always wore a suit and tie, which never showed the dog and cat fur or other undesirable outputs that frequently adorned my outfits. He understood the gastrointestinal tract on a cellular level and could recite, in exquisite detail, his most recent work on promotility agents in the canine intestine. He could be relied upon to ask ponderous, challenging questions at grand rounds, regardless of subject, and had mastered a quizzical frown he employed while the quivering resident answered. His knowledge was awesome, but his focus was theoretical. I was alone in trying to decode disease for Fritz's scared, ingenuous owner.

Ms. Whitney returned to the hospital later that day and, on sight, I had no doubt that she would do anything to save her dog. She came alone, no supportive friend, roommate, or partner, no protective parent. And it was her solitude, more than her designer jeans and white T-shirt, or her panicky grip on a Coach purse, that told me what Fritz was worth to her. She was alone in her love for this dog and, in turn, that love made her less alone.

She was petite—slim in the gaunt, brittle way of girls in their early twenties trying hard to be liked. I wanted to believe that we were nothing alike, that she was a daughter of privilege, living an easy life in a Rittenhouse Square apartment with her pampered dog, but I understood her desperation to save Fritz; I could barely imagine the desolation of life without Monty.

Fritz slumped listlessly on her lap. He'd summoned a dispirited tail wag when he first saw her, but he now looked miserable. She spoke softly to him. She gently laid her mouth close to his ear, urging him to keep fighting.

"I'll give you some time," I said, lingering awkwardly at the door before I stepped outside. I didn't know how to soothe the anguish I read on her face as she held the weight of her dog's illness in her arms.

I headed to the fourth-floor clinical pathology lab to check on Fritz's blood results. I wanted to know what his pancreatitis meant for the rest of his body. My instinct said it wasn't going to be good. Heading up the stairs I met Jean, a friend and senior resident, also on her way to the lab. We climbed the stairs chatting about our cases.

"How're things going?" Jean asked.

"Urgh, I picked up a difficult case this morning. A young dachshund with bad pancreatitis. I expect he'll be in the ICU by tonight. His ultrasound was ugly; he's already got fluid in his belly."

"Tough case. How's his owner?"

"That's the worst bit. She's young and really emotional, and she doesn't get how sick her dog is. I don't know how she'll react when I tell her he's getting worse."

"She's probably really scared," Jean said. "She might not have been through this kind of thing before."

I nodded. "He's probably sick because of a hot dog she fed him."

"Poor thing, she must feel terrible," Jean said.

"I feel worse for Fritz. Who's stupid enough to feed their twelve-pound dog a hot dog?"

"I know, but we always see the worst of the worst, and most people don't have a clue. They think dogs can eat anything. And some dogs can."

Our voices echoed off the flat gray of the stairwell. The familiar beep of a pager sounded somewhere below us. We reached the basket for completed lab reports and began searching for our patients' names.

"Not good." Jean handed me a sheet with Fritz's name in the top left corner.

"Everything looks worse," I said, noting his rising liver enzymes and falling blood proteins, both indicating that his body was taking a bad hit. His CBC showed that his white cell count was continuing to climb and his blood was no longer clotting normally; a dangerous combination suggesting the development of SIRS—systemic inflammatory response syndrome—a nasty acronym that might signal the beginning of a downward spiral I couldn't halt. I pointed to his coagulation profile. "He's heading to ICU," I said.

"Looks like it," Jean groaned. "Who are you on with?"

"Goldman," I replied.

"Better keep him in the loop; he hates cases transferring without him knowing."

I responded with a grunt and pulled out my pager. The bureaucratic hurdles I needed to jump to get Fritz into the ICU would occupy the next several hours of my day.

"Fancy a drink later?" Jean asked.

"You must've read my mind," I replied.

"I'll see what Gina and Mark are up to. Maybe we can head to the White Dog after work."

"Jean, you're a lifesaver." I headed down the stairwell with renewed determination.


In the hierarchy of consents needed to move Fritz into the ICU, his owner was at the bottom. Goldman's support was vital for my patient's smooth passage through the doors of the critical care unit. Luckily, after reviewing Fritz's lab results, he agreed that the dog's condition warranted the high-level treatment the ICU would provide. The next step was to convince the senior ICU clinician that Fritz needed to be admitted. My success was dependent on who was on duty, the caseload, and the number of animals expected to arrive after surgical procedures.

I was welcomed into the ICU by the competing bleeps of ECG monitors, fluid pump alarms, and blood pressure monitors. Unlike the hectic bustle of the ER, the ICU had a hushed, somber air, even during the most harried of resuscitation efforts. I stood in the doorway and surveyed the territory before stepping over the threshold. There were two large oxygen cages stacked one on top of the other close to the door. Each was big enough to house a medium-sized dog, and could be partitioned for cats or small dogs. Next to the oxygen cages were two dog runs for the biggest patients, one of which Hercules had occupied. Adjacent to the runs was a wall of various-sized cages for smaller patients. I pictured Fritz in one of these, and wanted to get him there as soon as possible.

A metal table in front of the oxygen cages was the place for the most critical patients: those needing mechanical ventilation or one-on-one nursing care. The ICU staff, residents, and clinicians saw a case of this severity as a challenge, a test of skill, a battle to be fought and won, but I knew it was often the last stop before a final resting place, somewhere I didn't want my patients to end up.

I felt a heightened anticipation. I was about to be questioned about my treatment choices, diagnostic plan, and case management by the senior ICU clinician, and the vet working that day was known for her uncompromising standards. In her unit, crying was more commonly due to her harsh appraisal of clinical acumen than a result of a patient's demise.

I'd memorized Fritz's lab values, and I silently inventoried my treatment decisions.

I stepped into the unit. "Dr. Roberts? Do you have a moment? I was hoping to transfer a case to the ICU today."

"Dr. Fincham, how can I be of assistance?"

My heart rate escalated to match the rapid tracing of an ECG I could see behind her head. "I have a canine patient with pancreatitis. I'm worried he's developing SIRS and might be going into DIC."

"Is that how you present a case?" she asked. "I expect more from a medicine resident."

"Sorry, yes, of course." I'd already screwed up, and I'd uttered only a sentence. "Fritz is a three-year-old male, neutered miniature dachshund. He was presented to the emergency room yesterday for an acute onset of vomiting, anorexia, and depression."

I continued to describe Fritz's condition, trying to communicate my growing concerns. I couldn't tell what Dr. Roberts was thinking. Her expression rarely changed with her mood. Her eyebrows typically remained in a serious line, and her laugh was a peculiar thing forced through her lips at unpredictable times.

"I was hoping that after Fritz finishes visiting with his owner we can transfer him directly to the ICU."

"Is his owner on board with the plan?" Dr. Roberts asked.

"She wants to do everything, and finances aren't an issue. I don't think it will be a problem."

"Of course, we have to get the owner's approval first, don't we, Dr. Fincham? But in principle, it would seem appropriate to transfer Fritz's care to the ICU."

"Great. Thank you." My instant relief at her decision sent me scurrying to the door of the unit. "I'll be back as soon as I can."

"I'll let Donna know so she can set up a cage. How are his jugulars?"

I hesitated. The integrity, or otherwise, of the two large, easily accessible veins running down Fritz's neck could influence our treatment options. The jugular veins were the only vessels suitable for the placement of the large catheters essential for monitoring hydration and delivering multiple fluid types, including intravenous nutrition, at one time. They were also, however, the veins most commonly used for drawing blood with a needle and syringe, which, in a sick patient with poor clotting ability and inflamed blood vessels, could quickly cause sufficient damage to render them unsuitable for catheter placement.

Fritz's veins were a problem. The consequence of his adorably short and twisted legs—apart from the multiple orthopedic problems they posed—was the roly-poly, awkward veins that ran down them. He had the type of blood vessels that were repellent to catheter placement or blood draws. That morning I'd noted that his leg veins were blown, his front leg catheter was tenuous, and one of his jugulars had already been damaged by venipuncture for blood sampling.

"One still looked good this morning," I said.

"I hope so. If not, life will be much more difficult."

I gave her a tight nod of agreement and headed to the stairs. I didn't want to answer any more questions until Fritz was safely in the unit.

I knocked on the exam room door, not waiting for a reply before stepping inside. Fritz's owner looked smaller and younger than I'd remembered, and Fritz looked ready for the ICU. I noticed that his chest was rising and falling with a deliberate effort.

"Sorry I took so long," I said. "I was reviewing Fritz's new lab results."

"I didn't notice. We've just been hanging out, haven't we, Fritzy?" His tail flickered against her leg. "That's a good sign, right? He must be feeling better if he's wagging his tail."

"I think he's just responding to the sound of your voice," I replied. "I'm very worried about Fritz. I think that his condition is getting worse."

"I don't understand. He seems fine, and the doctor in the emergency room told me he'd go home in a day or two."

"Fritz isn't going home yet. I know how worried you are about him, and how much you want him home with you, but pancreatitis is a very serious disease, and it can sometimes get worse no matter what we do. Despite doing everything we can, he's not showing any improvement. I think we should move him to the intensive care unit."

"'Intensive care unit'? But that's where the really sick dogs go, right? He only ate a hot dog; he can't be that sick."

A familiar frustration flushed my cheeks. I wanted to get Fritz to the ICU, to focus on medicine, and not on his owner's emotional distress.

"Fritz's best chance is if he goes to the ICU where he can be monitored more closely and receive additional treatment that we can't give in the wards."

"Like what?" she asked.

"He looks like he's having a hard time breathing, and in the ICU we can supplement his oxygen to make things easier for him."

"He usually breathes like this when he's excited. I think he's just excited to see me."

I dropped my gaze. It was easier to look at Fritz struggling to breathe than it was to meet his owner's eyes. "He doesn't look very excited at the moment," I said. "I'd like to get him to the ICU as soon as possible; that way we can see what's going on and decide what to do next. Okay?"

Fritz's owner lifted him to her chest and rested her chin on his head. Her tears rolled down his flank. He raised his nose to rest on her shoulder. His front leg, cheerfully wrapped in bright blue vet wrap, was sticking out awkwardly due to the IV catheter. It was a small movement, a sick dog seeking comfort from the person who loved him the most, but it took me outside my irritation, and beyond my doubts at my ability to help Fritz and his owner. It reminded me of Monty, and how, when he sensed that I was upset, he would sit on my lap while my tears fell onto his black coat.

"You can take him," she said, without loosening her grip. "I don't care how much it costs. I want Fritzy back. Do whatever you need to."

I lifted Fritz gently out of her arms and felt the slightest resistance when I took him from her. I should've made her wait for the new estimate from the financial department, but I didn't have the courage; it felt ugly and unpleasant to leave her to sit alone while I took Fritz to the ICU. I didn't stop her when she accompanied us to the door of the exam room.

Once in the ICU, I placed Fritz on the central treatment table, and instantly technicians, residents, and the senior clinician surrounded him. His veins were evaluated, vital signs checked, and blood pressure and oxygenation status obtained. I could barely see my patient through the melee of white coats and blue scrubs.

The moment I placed him on the table, I became obsolete in Fritz's care, although I would remain his primary doctor and the main contact for his owner. In the ICU I was merely an internal medicine resident, superseded by a rank of critical care doctors and technicians. I caught the attention of the resident long enough to tell her to page me if they needed me, before I headed back to the wards.

An hour later, I returned to the ICU. Fritz was in the oxygen cage; my concern about his breathing had been well founded. His lungs were filling with fluid and cells. His disease had moved into the territory of acronyms—SIRS (systemic inflammatory response syndrome) and ARDS (acute respiratory distress syndrome) had been added to his problem list. If we couldn't get a handle on the devastating inflammation in his body, he was likely to develop MODS (multiple organ dysfunction syndrome) and DIC (disseminated intravascular coagulation). And death would become inevitable.

Fritz lay in the back of the cage. Even in the enriched air, his chest moved with an exaggerated force, his flooded lungs trying to capture sufficient oxygen. Through the faintly scratched Plexiglas cage door I could see the results of his hour in the ICU. He was dwarfed by the tangle of leads and lines that ran to and from his body. His essential dogginess lessened with each patch of hair clipped for ultrasound, catheter placement, and blood draw. He was still a dog, but I wasn't sure if he was still Fritz.

I wouldn't be going out for drinks that night. Even though there was little I could do, I would spend as long as I could in the ICU before going home, where I expected my pager and my anxiety would keep me awake. As much as his care was now out of my hands, I still felt an urgent need to stand watch, imagining that he would continue breathing only as long as I kept my eyes on the labored rise and fall of his chest.

"Dr. Fincham?" I turned to find Dr. Roberts standing behind me. "We got an arterial line in, quite an achievement, and here's his blood gas. I wanted to see what you think."

She handed me the small strip of paper that revealed exactly how badly Fritz's lungs were doing. I looked at the numbers and reached for my calculator, hoping that my fumbling among the pens, hair, white tape, and other detritus at the bottom of my pocket would buy a minute for me to remember the formula I needed. It was a test. Dr. Roberts had already calculated the alveolar to arterial (A–a) oxygen gradient, which assessed how much oxygen was passing into the bloodstream, and therefore the severity of damage to the delicate permeable membrane of the alveolar walls. It would've been the first thing she did when the machine spat out the results. The formula for the A–a gradient was complicated, and given that Fritz was living in an oxygen cage, I knew it was abnormal.

The calculation was an exercise in academic medicine; the number wasn't going to change Fritz's treatment plan. But by calculating the gradient correctly my status in the ICU would incrementally increase.

I tried out the formula that came into my head. "Forty-four?"

"Are you asking me or telling me, Dr. Fincham?"

"Telling you. The A–a gradient is forty-four, which is abnormal. Fritz's lung function is decreased."

"Very good, and what does that mean for your patient?"

I looked at the small black and tan dachshund lying on a sunny baby blanket in the white noise of the oxygen cage. *He's going to die*, I thought.

"If he doesn't improve, then the only option will be to put him on the ventilator," I said.

"I agree. Have you discussed this with his owner?"

"No. He wasn't breathing this badly the last time we spoke. I can call her, but I think she will want to do everything."

I watched Fritz struggle to breathe, the movement of his chest a deliberate, conscious effort, his abdomen expanding and contracting with the force of each breath. His head was raised in an awkward position, with his neck extended.

"Do you think putting him on the ventilator is the right thing to do?" I asked.

"We don't have a choice. If this owner wants to save her dog it's the only option."

"But if we put him on the ventilator what are his chances of coming off it again and recovering?"

I was surprised to hear myself ask the question. I knew the answer; his prognosis was poor. While placing him under anesthesia and having a machine force oxygen into his lungs would help improve his blood oxygen level, it would do nothing to help the severe, cascading inflammation that was the root of the problem. Using the ventilator was our only chance of keeping him alive, but this chance—when we couldn't control the pancreatitis that continued to rage through his body—was slight.

"It's not our decision to make," Dr. Roberts replied. "And without ventilation he won't make it through the night. If we can give him enough time for his pancreatitis to resolve and his lung function to improve, he stands a good chance of making it home. I think he deserves that chance, don't you?"

I paused, unsure how, or if, I was expected to answer her question.

Fritz was a young dog; he had a potentially curable disease with no long-term consequences, and an owner with apparently limitless finances.

Didn't he deserve a chance? My gut told me that no matter how many catheters we placed, drugs we administered, or dollars we spent, Fritz was out of chances.

If this was the case, then was it right to put him and his owner through escalating invasive treatments? We had a choice to make. We didn't have to keep going. But the only other option was euthanasia.

Did Fritz feel like he was suffocating?

Was the inflammation in his abdomen causing pain that we weren't controlling?

Was the constant hum of the oxygen generator stressful?

I would never know how Fritz felt.

His owner would dictate his care, and I knew she would try anything to save this piece of her heart, regardless of his suffering. But when did the act of saving her dog become selfish?


By the time I got home the ventilator had been set up, the on-call resident paged, and the anesthetic drugs calculated. I no longer needed to stand watch over each of Fritz's breaths; now a machine would be breathing for him. Sitting on the couch with Monty curled on my lap, I replayed the events of the day. I tried to pinpoint the moment Fritz had taken his downturn, and questioned the decisions I'd made, wondering how I could have stopped his decline. I was angry that I'd failed my patient and worried that I'd missed an opportunity to interrupt the spiraling cascade that had led him to the ventilator. I'd failed to stand up to his disease and the invasive treatments. A line had been crossed.

"I'll never do that to you, I promise," I whispered to Monty, feeling the vibration of his purr against my body. No matter how much I needed him in my life, I vowed that I'd never subject him to the extremes of intensive care. But did I really know?

I didn't sleep that night, haunted by Fritz on a ventilator, Monty on a ventilator, Fritz dying, Monty dying—dangerously blurring the line between my personal and professional life.

The next morning, I arrived in the ICU to learn that Fritz's respiratory function had continued to decline overnight. His ventilator settings had needed constant tweaking to match his need for oxygen. I didn't want to examine him; he was absent, but his body was invaded—veins and arteries catheterized, an endotracheal tube securing access to his airway through his mouth, a nasogastric tube suctioning stomach contents, a urinary catheter accessing his bladder, and a rectal temperature probe.

Fritz lay swaddled in tubes and cables, sung to by the constant mechanical beep of his machines. His life had been reduced to rows of numbers, boxes filled in on a grid. The steps taken to save him had changed his body, and the disease had taken its toll.

Overnight, pancreatitis had spread through his body like an uncontrollable fire, and his blood vessels had become engulfed. The delicate, porous barrier that usually regulated the flow of fluid to and from tissues was damaged and ragged. Fritz had become a swollen, gelatinous version of the dog I remembered. Fluid had seeped into his lungs and vital organs, hastening the advancement of multi-organ failure. The fire had engulfed his foundations.

There was nothing more to do. His lungs were saturated, his kidneys failing. Within hours, regardless of what we did, he would be dead. I didn't know if inside his bloated body a part of Fritz still lingered, but if there was any chance that an enduring sentience remained I wanted to release it. To give him back the dignity he'd been stripped of in the last hours of his life. But first I had to obtain his owner's consent for euthanasia.

I picked up the phone, "Good morning, Ms. Whitney, it's Dr. Fincham."

"How's Fritz. Is he alive? Is he breathing on his own?"

"Fritz made it through the night, but—"

"Thank goodness, I've been so worried. I knew he'd make it for me, he's such a fighter."

"But," I continued, "unfortunately, despite everything we've done, his condition has continued to deteriorate." I waited for a reply but there was silence. "Can you come to the hospital as soon as possible?"

"Why?" Her voice sounded breathless and thin. "Is he dying? Is he dying right now? Why didn't you call sooner?"

*Because it wouldn't have changed anything.* "Fritz is alive, but he's very sick. His lungs and now his other internal organs, including his kidneys and liver, are failing. We need to think about how much further to go."

"What are you saying? That I should give up? Is that what you're telling me?"

"It's not giving up. We've done everything, and there is nothing more we can do. I think it's time to consider euthanasia."

"He's going to make it. I know he is. I'm not giving up on him, no matter what. I promised him that I would never leave him."

"I know this is hard, but Fritz is dying. I'm worried that he's suffering, and we can help him with that. You could be with him, and hold him. We can make it very peaceful."

"No. No. You can't make me kill my dog." I took a breath and asked her to meet me at the hospital. She agreed, and while I waited for the page to tell me she'd arrived I could only hope that she'd change her mind.

Fifteen minutes later, I met Fritz's owner in the lobby and accompanied her to the ICU. There was nothing more to say. She would not, or could not, change her mind, and inside the unit I stepped aside for the critical care resident to explain the compromise they'd reached.

"We're going to keep Fritz anesthetized and turn off the ventilator," the resident said. "Without the machine breathing for him his tissues will quickly become starved of oxygen."

"But there's a chance he could wake up, right? He might start breathing on his own and be okay."

"I'm very sorry, but I don't think Fritz is going to wake up," the resident continued. "His lungs are so damaged that even if he does breathe on his own, he won't be able to take in enough oxygen."

"You're telling me he's going to die?"

"Ms. Whitney, I'm so sorry. We've done everything we possibly can. There's nothing more we can do."

"He's going to die, then?" Fritz's owner asked again.

"Are you sure you won't consider euthanasia?" I asked. "You could hold him. Fritz wouldn't suffer at all."

"No. I'm gonna give him a chance. I won't let you kill my dog."

I stepped back, silently hating her and her inability to do what I thought was right.

"It's okay, Ms. Whitney," the ICU resident stepped in. "We'll proceed as planned. I'm going to turn off the monitors so they don't distract us."

The monitors would alarm when Fritz's blood pressure, oxygen levels, and heart rate dropped. We didn't need to be alerted. It was the order of death.

Fritz's owner stood at his head and the resident flanked the ventilator. I took another step back.

The resident leaned forward. "Tell me when you're ready."

Fritz's owner's denial turned into a terrible sobbing. Her body shook and she wrapped her arms tightly around herself. "I don't think I can do this," she said. "I can't lose him; he means everything to me."

"I know how hard this must be," the ICU resident said. "But you're doing the right thing. Fritz isn't going to get better."

Her sobbing rose to a wail of assent.

The ventilator huffed its last breath, and for a moment nothing changed. Fritz didn't move or take a breath. His tongue, stuck at an awkward angle from his mouth, remained pink. His owner grabbed his swollen paw, urgently whispering to him to breathe. I held my breath. I knew what was coming, what the process of dying looked like. But I felt no relief when Fritz began a gasping respiratory pattern. Each heave was a reminder of my failure. Anger built behind my larynx, and while Fritz continued to gasp, his tongue turning the purple-blue of cyanosis, a sob grabbed at my throat.

I had witnessed the final breath of many animals, after administering euthanasia solution or during desperate resuscitation measures. But I'd never experienced the impotence I felt watching Fritz suffocate. I would not cry in the ICU. It was frowned upon. But the stifled sobs rippled through me, trying to escape. I turned away. I walked to the door of the ICU, stepped through, and closed it behind me.

# CHAPTER FIVE

# Zeke

By 2003, I'd become as accustomed as possible to the putrid soup of Philadelphia summers. Nevertheless, I still found the rotten, swelling heat difficult to deal with. Walking home from the hospital at night, I passed brick walls of apartment buildings that radiated the sun they'd stored from the blazing day; the streets might as well have been lined with pizza ovens. The trash cans dotting each block stained the air with the odor of decaying food and dirty diapers.

My life was dictated by the academic calendar. School started in September and finished in July, and internships and residencies began and ended in June. I was nearing the end of my residency and, rather than fireplaces in cozy British pubs and windblown rain seeping between narrow gaps in my clothing, I was greeted by languid, fetid heat after each shift. A year was marked by the graduation of students and the completion of training programs, not the bang of fireworks or the promise of New Year's resolutions.

I'd imagined that my life would be perpetually measured in school years, accumulating board certification, then a PhD, then a bibliography of first-authored papers in scientific journals. But the happiness that I'd anticipated would come from singularly pursuing veterinary medicine ebbed into the porous ground of my discontent.

I had no real home. Life in America still seemed temporary. And my English friends had boyfriends I'd never met, listened to music I'd never hear, and told stories I didn't understand. Unsurprising, then, that by the end of my residency I'd acquired a new family—my three cats, Monty, Fred, and Harry—to help soften the edge of my loneliness.

Fred had arrived a little less than a year after Monty, about the time I was accepted for my residency. He was a three-month-old white kitten, with patches of striped brown tabby on his tail, sides, and ears. A technician at VHUP had found him clinging to her screen door. Facing the next two years in Philadelphia, I instantly decided that a new kitten was exactly what I—and Monty—needed, given the long hours I spent at the hospital. But Monty merely tolerated his frantic new companion. The cozy relationship I'd imagined between them never transpired.

Monty liked to sit on the windowsill watching birds, lounge on the hardwood floor in swaths of sun, and sleep at the foot of my bed. Fred did not. He preferred to chase imaginary bugs up and down the walls, find ingenious places to hide, and keep his distance from the human and feline members of his family.

A year later, about halfway through my residency, I adopted Harry to bridge the gap between Monty and Fred. He was an orange and white tabby, acquired by way of my resident mate Jean. He'd been evaluated for an unknown gastrointestinal disease, which had caused his previous owners to give him up to a rescue group. The problem turned out to be a penny lodged in his intestine, which was surgically removed. When I brought him home, Harry was a leggy, boisterous teenager, still with a hairless patch on his downy white belly clipped from surgery.

I called him my rock star; he greeted everyone, hopping onto laps regardless of whether consent had been granted, and leaving a powdering of orange and white fur on suit trousers, smart dresses, scrubs, and jeans without discrimination. His eyes were a peculiar sea-glass green, and his coat had the soft nap of a wild creature. He was my once-in-a-lifetime cat, the one all others would be compared to and found lacking. With Harry, I felt like the unpopular girl in school who'd landed the hottest boyfriend. Harry proved to be the perfect addition to my feline family. He was happy to curl up for a nap with Monty or chase Fred around the apartment. And my three cats were the perfect welcome-home after a long day at the hospital.

I had the notion, through veterinary school and my internship, that the senior clinicians I worked with were godlike. They were the people I aspired to be, the goal I might one day achieve. I thought that with an academic career, I could lose myself in microscopic minutiae, focused so intently on a single viewpoint that there would be no space for loneliness. But, with the passage of time, I came to realize that neither the study of infectious organisms and biochemical pathways, nor the number of journal articles authored, would bring the happiness I was seeking.

In the final months of my residency, echoes of confrontations with my resident mates and senior clinicians haunted my days in the hospital. I was furious that the gods I'd created in my mind were, in reality, made of the exact same cells, proteins, and molecules as I was. The end of my residency drew closer, and my decision to stay in academia or to leave became inescapable.

The point of combustion came on a Sunday. It had been a long weekend—the pick-ups from the emergency room were an array of bad diseases with worse prognoses. I was the senior resident on service and had taken the brunt of the transfers. By Sunday afternoon I was stationed in the ICU fighting to save a young dog from dying of protein-losing nephropathy (PLN)—a disease where the kidneys' filtration system is damaged by inflammation or infection. This injury causes large holes to form in the tightly regulated barrier of the kidney (glomerular) membrane, causing essential proteins to be lost into the urine. I had seen enough of the disease to know there was little I could do to alter the grave prognosis. My previous attempts at treatment had resulted in dogs drowning in the intravenous fluids I'd administered in an attempt to save their lives.

My patient was a two-year-old black, male Labrador retriever. The flat, recycled air of the ICU couldn't cool the anxiety that was rising between the nape of my neck and the collar of my white coat. The flimsy paper with my patient's most recent blood gas analysis that was stuck to my damp fingertips revealed what I most dreaded. The fluids I'd gingerly administered and fastidiously monitored had oozed into his lungs. Now there was nothing more I could do.

The senior internal medicine clinician on duty that weekend was a young, tall, friendly woman who I imagined to be better suited to a junior high school library than a veterinary ICU. She had blond hair, always tied back in a ponytail, and small features that crowded in the center of her face. I dreaded being on clinics with her. Her special topic of interest, which she would discuss at every opportunity, was Lyme disease, a tick-borne infection of growing reputation. The purported consequences ranged from PLN to seizures to heart failure.

"Dr. Fincham," she said from behind me. "I was just finishing up my rounds and wanted to check in." I turned to face her, and she looked down at the clipboard she always carried in the clinic. "How's Buddy?" She smiled encouragingly.

I shrugged.

"I didn't realize he'd moved to the ICU," she continued. "I was looking for you in wards."

"Sorry. I paged you earlier. I didn't like how he was breathing, so I moved him over midmorning."

If she'd been another senior clinician, I might have felt guilt at my lack of communication. Instead, I felt a defiant, childish triumph that my case had transferred without her knowledge.

"How are things going?" she asked.

"His blood gas looks bad, he's hypertensive, and I think he's developing pulmonary edema."

"Oh dear. Do you have him on anti-emetics?"

"Yes," I replied. *Of course I do.* "I started them yesterday, along with antacids."

She nodded. "Good."

*It's not good, though, is it?* I wanted to yell. *Look at this dog. He's two years old, and he's going to die. Why can't you help me?*

"Do we know the underlying cause of his protein-losing nephropathy?" she continued. "I was wondering if you'd considered infectious diseases?"

*Go on,* I thought, anger creeping from the base of my skull. *Tell me about your research on Lyme nephritis.* The indignation jolted along my jawbone with an electricity that bordered on excitement. *Tell me some esoteric fact about the pathogenesis of the infectious organism that won't make the slightest difference to my patient.*

"Yes," I answered. "The emergency doctor submitted a tick panel when he first presented. It was positive for Lyme."

"How exciting. Would his owners consider a kidney biopsy? I'm looking at some new tests we can use on tissue specimens to prove the causative relationship between the *Borrelia* organism and the lesions we are seeing in dogs with PLN."

*A kidney biopsy? An invasive procedure requiring general anesthesia in a dog who was dying.* A derisive laugh escaped.

For a second Dr. Wilson continued smiling. But then she looked down, her eyes welling with shocked sadness.

"I think it's a bit late for that," I said, my voice growing louder. "I don't think biopsying his kidney now is going to help, is it?" I figured she could have as much kidney for her experiments as she wanted in a few hours, when my patient was dead.

*I needed you to help me,* I wanted to say. *You've let me down. You're supposed to be better than me.*

I took a step backward, immediately feeling the weight of my disrespect in the shocked silence of the ICU. Remorse swept away my fury, but I was too proud to apologize, and instead I left with tears swarming to my eyes. I'd wanted to show that veterinary medicine wasn't only clinical trials and laboratory experiments. I'd wanted to bring down the gods I'd become disillusioned with. But I'd taken my frustration out on the wrong person and, in doing so, realized only a deeper anger with myself.

A meeting with the section chief the following morning, an official apology to the disrespected senior clinician, and my promise to behave more professionally could not seal the jagged cracks that had ripped through the vision of the future I'd been driving toward. My growing internal disillusionment had finally broken through the brittle carapace I had formed, and once it was out it could not be returned. It was this moment, more than any other, that determined my future in veterinary medicine.

Although I would complete my residency in a few months, I needed another year of study before I could take the board examinations and qualify as a veterinary internal medicine specialist. Most of my resident mates would be staying on at Penn, taking yearlong staff clinician positions to complete board certification before deciding on their next steps, but I would not be offered this chance. My growing ire had burned bridges, and it was time to move on.

For the first time since I'd resolved to become a veterinarian I had run out of path to blindly follow. I would be leaving academia at the end of my residency, and I didn't know what would come next. My visa was expiring, and I had to make the decision, yet again, to stay in the United States or return to the United Kingdom.

In the perfect plan I'd formulated, I was going to return to England with my board certification, ready to study for my PhD in veterinary immunology. I'd even decided that I'd work in the lab at my alma mater. But with my waning conviction that academic medicine was my future came the realization that England was no longer my home. The few friends I'd kept in touch with were scattered across the country, and private specialty practices were scarce. My loneliness couldn't be soothed by driving on the left or buying a lifetime supply of Marmite, and I had to acknowledge that my desire to return to my country of birth was less potent than I'd expected. My growing feline family tied me to the United States, but I felt a deep guilt over remaining so far from my family in England.

It was an uncomfortable decision, but I applied for positions in private specialty practices on the East Coast. I ignored the warnings of my senior clinicians that it would be hard to study for boards while working, and that I still had case reports to submit. I found a practice in Baltimore that seemed like a good fit, and that offered me a position to start at the end of my residency. By stepping away from the university I knew it was unlikely that I'd return. You were either in or out. I understood what I was giving up, but the more I'd learned, the more invested I'd become in the animals I treated. Greater than the science and the method, the discovery of my patients, the revelation of their temperaments, and the understanding of their relationships with their owners had gripped me. In private practice, I could focus on this aspect of veterinary medicine without the procedural bureaucracy of academia getting in the way.

Despite my trepidation at leaving the protective custody of academia, graduating to the real world was thrilling. I bought my first car. I rented an apartment in a converted warehouse in Baltimore—with central air—and I could finally afford cable. My new Fells Point neighborhood was right on the harbor, in a historic part of the city. It was the perfect place for my freshly liberated life. The cobblestone streets and pubs on every corner reminded me of home, and I could walk to enough independent shops and restaurants to put my increased salary to use. The one-bedroom had plenty of room for Monty, Fred, and Harry, who could chase imaginary bugs and watch seabirds all day, while also finding time to locate the best kitchen cupboard to sleep in. It was a twenty-minute drive to my new clinic in the suburbs, and I found a local radio station that played indie music close to my own taste. I worked just four days a week, and my vacation schedule wasn't determined by the academic calendar. I felt free.

One of the first patients I treated in Baltimore was Zeke, a decidedly American-sized cat who easily weighed sixteen pounds. The hospital was newly built and situated in a small retail park of blandly similar buildings. The gray uniformity of the interior echoed the exterior, but its most attractive feature was that it was clean: The physical assault of thousands of dog paws, millions of animal hairs, and a splattering of bodily secretions had not accumulated to any significant degree.

At our first meeting, Zeke sat hunched uncomfortably on the examination table, more ovoid than cat-shaped. We were in a small consulting room that offered, through tinted windows, a banal view of a dirt lot. Zeke had arrived at the clinic after the bloodwork his family veterinarian had run that morning showed severely elevated liver enzymes. These results, along with other indicators of liver failure, warranted his immediate transfer for intensive care.

Zeke was a silver-brown tabby, and his coloring initially made the yellow hue of his skin difficult to discern upon examination. He was jaundiced, or icteric; a yolky yellow pigment had been deposited in his skin due to the abnormal processing of bilirubin by his liver. When I assessed the inside of Zeke's ears and the sparsely haired stripes running from his ears to his eyes, the accumulation of bilirubin was so severe that it looked like he'd been colored with a highlighter. His gums were tinged orange, like coral lipstick, rather than a healthy pink. And the whites of his eyes—evaluated by lifting his eyelid to examine the sclera—were pure yellow.

Such findings on physical examination were small triumphs. To detect with my hands and eyes an abnormality later confirmed by lab tests, X-rays, or ultrasound was thrilling. There were times I still felt shaky, but the mechanistic ritual of the exam, performing the same sequence of movements on every dog and cat every time, provided a bedrock of experience I'd come to trust.

"When did you first notice something was wrong?" I asked Zeke's owner, Mrs. James. She was a short, fair-haired woman I guessed was in her late fifties. Her wedding band was overly snug and worn. Her clothing was unremarkable: a knee-length skirt and nondescript sweater that would suit a job in an office cubicle. A nervous tightness gripped the skin around her eyes, and she fiddled with the pleats of her skirt, her ring, and her hair.

"He seemed fine until a day or so ago," she replied. "He vomited three times yesterday, or maybe the day before. Yellow bile. No food. He does that sometimes, but today he seemed like he didn't feel good, so I took him in to my vet."

"When did he last eat?"

"We put fresh food out every day, so this morning, I think."

"Did you see him eat?" I refined my question.

"No, but he likes to sneak a bite when I'm not looking. I don't always pay that much attention."

"When was the last time you saw him at the bowl?"

"Come to think of it, not for the last week or so. Sometimes my husband feeds him, sometimes I do. I suppose his bowl's been pretty full since last weekend, but I thought my husband was topping it up. We fill the bowl and then Zeke eats as much as he wants, which is usually all of it, isn't it, Zeke? He loves his food." Her hand fretted on Zeke's back, his fur growing darker and flatter from the heat of her palm.

"He loves treats," she said. "He'll do anything for them. He'll even beg on his back legs like a dog if I ask him. That's about the only activity he'll do, though. Sleeping and eating, those are his favorite things."

*Typical cat,* I thought, picturing my own three felines who were probably napping on the couch at that moment, but were always instantly and demandingly awake an hour before feeding time.

Each species presents unique challenges to a veterinarian, but cats, true to their inscrutable nature, can be particularly difficult. The fear induced by a visit to the vet's office only compounds the problem. Nervous cats may refuse to walk, slink skittishly around the perimeter of the exam room, or hide in the darkest corner of their carrier, which can make assessing their gait and neurologic function challenging. Their heart and respiration rate, body temperature, and even blood glucose levels can become elevated due to the release of stress hormones, and these parameters can be almost useless diagnostic tools in certain cats.

The cats who manifest their fright with aggression are formidable patients, as Tiger had already taught me. Fred, my own mild-mannered but nervous kitten, became a screaming ball of claws and teeth when I took him in for his neuter. He pulled out his intravenous catheter while recovering from anesthesia, spraying himself and the walls of his cage with blood while hissing and swatting at anyone who tried to help. I felt like an embarrassed parent with a toddler in a tantrum. "He's nothing like this at home," I wanted to say, imagining I had some control over my pet's behavior.

Despite humans' centuries-long association with cats, it has been only in the past one hundred years that the veterinary profession has considered feline patients. It took the Industrial Revolution and the development of the motorcar for veterinarians to turn their attention away from horses and to smaller companion animals. Cats have evolved little, if at all, over this period, but our attitude toward them has radically shifted. Kidney transplantation has become a routine procedure for specialized feline surgeons; and specifically formulated medications for cats and the array of food in pet stores attest to the massive social and economic change the domestic cat has undergone in less than a century.

Cats are now the most popular pet in the United States, with the ASPCA reporting that 74 to 96 million cats are owned as pets, compared to 70 to 80 million dogs. But they lag significantly behind their canine counterparts where veterinary care is concerned. Given that the act of getting a cat to the vet can leave you exhausted, bloody, and smelling of excrement before even leaving the house, it is unsurprising that cat owners are reluctant to take them in for preventive care. For cats, a waiting room of barking, panting dogs, being wrestled out of their carriers, the indignities of rectal temperature taking, and the further invasion of blood sampling or vaccine administration explain their objections.

Unfortunately, avoiding preventive care means that treatable diseases may not be detected until it's too late for effective treatment. And cats, particularly if they live in multi-cat households, can obscure the signs of disease that might alert us to a problem sooner. Litter boxes are kept far from human activity, so toileting behavior is rarely witnessed. Food is left in free-feed bowls, so consumption is not quantified. And cats naturally spend a large portion of their day lying around doing nothing—how can an owner tell, then, if lounging is simply enjoying the sun or is a result of weakness or lethargy? It is often only when their behavior becomes inconvenient—vomiting on a favorite pair of shoes, or peeing on the clean laundry—that veterinary attention is sought.

Although these problems with providing veterinary care for cats are easily identifiable, their solutions are less obvious. There is no easy, foolproof method of getting a reluctant cat into a carrier, into the car, and to the vet's office. Home visits can alleviate the stress, but it's not possible to take X-rays, perform extensive diagnostics, or pursue intensive treatment at home. The American Association of Feline Practitioners' Cat Friendly Practice initiative was designed to make vet visits more comfortable for cats. Separate waiting rooms and treatment areas for cats and dogs and the use of calming cat pheromones have been identified as ways to alleviate feline stress at the vet, but these measures are beneficial only if our patients make it into the office.

Zeke's previous medical record showed that his visits to the vet had been sporadic, and I didn't know how he'd behaved the last time he'd gone in for a broken claw, but his highlighter-hued skin justified his attitude in my examination room that day. The bilirubin coursing through his bloodstream and depositing in his tissues was likely causing nausea. Toxins normally excreted by his failing liver were accumulating in his brain, causing changes in the delicately balanced chemistry that could result in depression and coma.

"I think Zeke hasn't been eating well for longer than we think," I said.

"But he seemed fine a day or two ago," Mrs. James replied.

"I know this seems out of the blue, but Zeke most likely has a condition called hepatic lipidosis, which can occur suddenly. We usually see it in overweight cats who stop eating, sometimes because of stress, a change in food, or another disease."

"Zeke doesn't get stressed. He's so laid-back. He spends most of his time lounging around."

"I don't mean *stress* the way we think of it. Stress for a cat could mean a visitor coming to stay, a new cat in the neighborhood, or even moving the furniture around."

"I can't think of anything that's changed. Our routine's been the same."

I nodded. "We don't always know why some cats develop hepatic lipidosis."

I explained how, when an overweight cat stops eating, energy is released from fat stores, rather than from food. Mobilized fat travels to the liver for processing, but instead of being metabolized, the lipids become trapped within liver cells. The liver cells fill with fat, like bloated balloons. Just like a hamburger and fries for lunch makes you sluggish in the afternoon, the fat stops the liver cells from working properly. The liver starts to fail, suppressing appetite further, and more fat is mobilized and deposited in the struggling cells. A vicious cycle ensues. Ultimately, the liver gives up, and death from liver failure can result.

Mrs. James's expression became progressively stricken while I described the reason for Zeke's illness. Her hand was motionless on his back.

"Are you saying he could die?" she asked.

"Some cats with severe lipidosis die from the disease, but I'm hopeful that if we can get food into Zeke we can start reversing the liver failure."

Relief flashed in her eyes. "I was saying to my husband that we should try a different food. I thought he was just being picky; you know how cats are."

"Unfortunately it's not that straightforward. Most of the time when cats start to get picky about their food it's because something is making them not feel good."

"But maybe he got tired of his food. We usually feed him the same kibble; maybe he wants more variety."

"I know it might seem that way, but Zeke is too sick to want to eat on his own right now, and we need to make sure that he's getting enough calories to reverse the damage to his liver."

"I'm sure I can get him eating at home; he did eat a treat this morning. I can hand-feed him, right, Zeke?"

Mrs. James's sudden optimism was disconcerting, but not unfamiliar. She had transferred her grief and anxiety over Zeke's illness into a more manageable concern. My words about liver failure and death were eclipsed by the more pressing matter of a visit to the pet store to purchase new cat food.

The clinical reality, however, was more urgent and less easily addressed. Without adequate nutrition in the next twenty-four to forty-eight hours, it was likely that Zeke would die from irreversible liver failure. To rely on his appetite was too big a risk to take. The only way to ensure we could meet his caloric needs was to place a feeding tube.

Zeke's feeding tube placement would be straightforward. Despite the need for a scalpel, suture material, and other instruments that usually made my hands shake, I'd performed the procedure enough times to find a grip-stilling confidence. I would ease a thin, flexible tube through a small incision in Zeke's neck and into his esophagus. It was satisfying to think of his liver recovering with each liquid feeding—the fat bubbles deflating; the cells returning to their normal size and to their work, processing toxins and bilirubin.

"Zeke's condition is too serious for him to go home," I said. "He's going to be in the hospital for a few days."

"Are you sure there's nothing we can do for him at home? He's never slept a night out of the house. I don't think he'll like being in the hospital, will you, Zeke?"

Zeke was motionless, his body hunched and his head resting on the table.

"If I thought there was something you could do at home, I would tell you," I said. "But Zeke's liver is so badly damaged that he needs hospital care right now. Without it I don't think he'll make it."

She nodded and smiled briefly. "I thought you'd say that. It's not just up to me, though; I'll have to call my husband at work. Let him know what's going on. How much is this going to cost?"

"I'll have my staff bring in an estimate." I paused. "I also wanted to mention that Zeke will need tube feeding when he goes home."

"He will? How does that work?"

"Don't worry about it at the moment; let's get Zeke home with you first. But we'll give you full instructions when it's time for his discharge. Usually the feedings are two to three times a day, and take twenty to thirty minutes each."

"How do people do that? We both work full-time. I don't know how we'll manage that."

I tried to look reassuring. I wanted to treat Zeke; he had a potentially curable disease with no long-term consequences—a rare occurrence in the world of small-animal internal medicine.

"I know it sounds overwhelming," I said. "But once you get into the routine it's quite straightforward."

Zeke's owner's face was difficult to read; her lips looked blanched in the fluorescent light of the examination room. She clasped the phone she'd pulled from her bag on mention of her husband. I wanted to add more words of reassurance, promise Zeke's recovery and return home, but I couldn't guarantee it. I stepped out of the room to plan his treatment and diagnostic course for the next twenty-four hours.

If Zeke survived his initial hospitalization, his prognosis was good. But some cats with hepatic lipidosis didn't eat for a month, or two, or even longer, and needed tube feeding every day until they began eating again. I thought of my routine, of how I was out of the house for fourteen or fifteen hours on workdays, and of how the time I spent with my cats was limited to sleeping in bed with the top sheet tent-pegged by feline bodies. How would I find time to blend and warm the food, flush the feeding tube, administer medications, and then patiently feed sixty milliliters of warmed, meaty gruel several times every day?

What and how we feed our animal companions is crucial to the bond we share with them. It is also big business, with the global pet food market estimated to be worth $74.8 billion in 2017. But only 150 years ago cats survived on what they caught, and dogs lived on household scraps, and, if particularly lucky, bread soaked in milk.

What we feed our pets is as much a lifestyle choice as what we eat ourselves. For some owners, feeding is a tangible, quantifiable measure of love. Our ideas of good cat and dog nutrition are influenced by our personal food preferences, advertising, and our ethical and philosophical beliefs. It is unsurprising, given the complex nature of our relationship with food, whether human or animal, that more than 54 percent of dogs and 59 percent of cats in the United States in 2016 were reportedly obese. And the link between obesity and disease in our pets is well documented. The catalog of health problems encountered by overweight cats and dogs includes shortened life expectancy, orthopedic problems, and metabolic diseases, including Zeke's hepatic lipidosis. Zeke's dietary habits had inevitably led him to my consulting room, but that was not a discussion I wanted to broach with Mrs. James in our first meeting.

My role was to get Zeke home. I understood what lay ahead for his owner, but I couldn't understand how the placement of a thin, flexible feeding tube might affect her relationship with Zeke, her husband, or the other unnamed people in her life.

I knew little about my client—only that she had an overweight cat, a husband, and a job. I knew what Zeke liked to eat and where he slept. I knew he liked to carry a small, balding toy mouse around the house, that he preferred water from the faucet, and that he'd stand on the kitchen counter demanding his after-dinner drink. I didn't know if his owner was squeamish about tubes and syringes and holes covered with bright bandages.

I didn't know if the smell of blended cat food would make her skip her own breakfast. I didn't know if her husband would help with feedings. Would he prepare the food? Go to Target to buy a designated blender? Would she lie to him about the cost of Zeke's treatment? These were questions beyond the scope of taking a history. But my success as Zeke's doctor was intimately connected to his treatment at home. I could get him through the next few days. I could recheck his bloodwork and body weight, adjust medications, and provide new feeding directions, but once he was out of the hospital, Zeke's recovery would depend on his owners.

I returned to the exam room twenty minutes later, after Mrs. James had approved the estimate. Zeke's large, striped body was awkwardly lumped across her knees. She scratched gently behind his ear, but the movement of his chest told me that he'd failed to summon a purr.

"We'll get treatments started right away," I said. "We'll place an intravenous catheter, begin fluids and medications, and run more tests to evaluate his liver. I'll call with an update once I have more information. Do you have any questions?"

"You're going to take good care of him, aren't you?"

"Of course. We'll do everything we can to get him home as soon as possible. I know how important he is to you."

"We want you to do whatever needs to be done. I don't know what we'd do if we lost him. He's our baby, aren't you, Zeke?" A flush of emotion spread from her eyes, and I realized that her earlier joviality had been a cover for the tears she was trying not to shed.

I scooped Zeke gently out of her lap.

Once Zeke and I returned to the treatment room, I pounced on the head technician, Shannon, and quickly relayed my diagnostic and treatment plan. I was accustomed to the bustling pace of Penn—supplies ready, techs awaiting instruction.

"Hang on," Shannon said. "You need to slow down." She was a few years older than me and had worked at the practice from its opening a year prior. Her engagement ring glinted in the fluorescent lights—a status symbol I considered impractical given the fur that must regularly get caught in its tiny prongs. She reminded me of Elisa, with a similar attention to her appearance, but with less sexual ferocity. She, nevertheless, ruled the internal medicine service with the same intimidating steel.

But, despite being the youngest and least experienced of the three-doctor internal medicine practice, I was no longer a trainee. I hadn't yet achieved board certification like my colleagues, but I craved the respect afforded to the other specialists.

"I can't get all these treatments down while you're talking so fast," she said, "and I have to finish with John's last case. You're going to have to wait."

I frowned. "But Zeke has hepatic lipidosis. He's really sick and we need to get started with him."

I watched impatience ripple across her jaw. "I know you're worried about your patient," she said, "but you have to give me some time."

"We need to check his blood-clotting to see if he needs a plasma transfusion before I can place his feeding tube, and he needs an ultrasound, maybe a liver aspirate, chest X-rays, and a blood gas." I checked each off on my fingers, which were vibrating with frustration.

"I know. But this isn't Penn. It's only me and Heather this afternoon, so you need to give me a break. Everyone has things they need me to do. Why don't you go and work on records, and I'll page you when we're ready for the ultrasound."

"And how long will that be?" I asked. She was treating me like a naughty child being sent to her room.

"An hour or so."

"I'll leave him here in his carrier, then?" I tried to keep my outrage from my voice.

"Sure, that's fine."

"See you soon, Zeke. We're going to take really good care of you," I said, leaving the treatment room before I could say something I'd regret.

The doctors' office was in the basement. The walls were an uninspiring cream, and the furniture gray, which matched the carpet. The air smelled new—fresh paint and the woodiness of plyboard. I was the only one to use the office; my colleagues preferred to type records and return phone calls at workstations in the treatment room.

At my desk I kicked off my new shoes. After three years of wearing scrubs and sneakers, I'd splurged on a new wardrobe I'd thought appropriate for a young, confident veterinarian. Sensible but fashionable. Tailored pants and colored shirts that fit under my white coat, with coordinating cute shoes, which I quickly realized were not designed for crawling around on all fours examining a Great Dane.

I was twenty-seven, regularly carded in bars, and still challenged by clients asking "Are you a real doctor?" or commenting "Wow, they train 'em young these days."

I'd decided that establishing my seniority was best achieved with wardrobe. And to some degree I'd been successful. However, I was still referred to as the "young one with the funny accent." I had yet to realize that tap dancing in my fancy shoes on the polished hospital floor, testing how fast I could spin down the hall on the wheeled office chair, and singing to my patients while performing ultrasounds were doing more damage than a wardrobe could repair.

While I regained the feeling in my toes, I stared at the wall where I wasn't permitted to affix anything. The cards and pictures I'd accumulated at Penn were reluctantly stored away. I opened Zeke's chart to begin typing his record. It was a disadvantage of leaving academia that the mundanity of writing subjective, objective, assessment, and plan (SOAP) notes; case summaries; and discharge instructions now fell to me, not a student.

I turned first to the page of serum chemistry results and looked down the column of three-letter acronyms, with their corresponding numbers, conveniently identified as high or low based on a comparison to the normal range.

Although Zeke's clinical picture most likely indicated hepatic lipidosis, I tested out the other possibilities on my list and felt a flop of hesitation. I knew the typical enzyme patterns associated with different types of liver disease, but not every patient followed the textbook, and I couldn't review my differentials with an attending clinician, or bounce the case off a resident mate. Maybe I'd missed the atypical presentation of an infection or tumor in Zeke's liver. *Don't chase zebras,* I reminded myself.

I would run the standard tests: an abdominal ultrasound to look at his liver, and a tiny ultrasound-guided-needle aspiration to ensure his hepatocytes looked under the microscope as I imagined them. I would continue monitoring his liver enzymes to ensure they decreased, and add broad-spectrum antibiotics in case of a lurking infection. The plan was familiar, but there was no safety net. I could—and had to—practice medicine the way I wanted, and develop my own clinical intuition rather than rely on someone else's.

"Hey, Suzy!"

I turned sharply. John, the head internal medicine specialist, stood in the doorway. Tall, with the slight stoop of a reluctant teenager embarrassed by his new height, he could summon an imposing de-meanor when pressed, but *goofy* usually came to mind when I thought of him. John had taught in London for a few years; he had been one of my lecturers at the Royal Veterinary College, before returning to the United States and joining this internal medicine practice.

"Hi, John. How's it going?" I fumbled my feet into the shoes dis-carded under my desk.

"Pretty good, just grabbing some lunch. I finished that ultrasound, so you're up next."

"Thanks. I'll get started. Would you be able to take a look at it with me? I haven't done many liver aspirates yet, and I'd really appre-ciate your help."

"I can take a look when I get back—not sure how long I'm going to be gone, though. I've got some records to write up and then a few more appointments, but I can help if I'm available."

I wanted to seem confident and competent, but I didn't trust my ultrasound skills. I'd watched hundreds of abdominal ultrasounds, peering over the radiologist's shoulder, trying to guess what the two-dimensional, monochrome image represented. Was it normal or ab-normal? Enlarged or shrunken? With someone else holding the probe I was good at identifying the changes. But with it in my hands, all I could reveal was a sea of unidentifiable structures.

John was no longer my teacher, and the priorities in private prac-tice were different. My entreaties were unlikely to be effective. Hours spent discussing cases or reviewing journal articles was time away from seeing cases—ultimately the only way the practice could sur-vive. Suppliers of medications and equipment didn't take IOUs, and the laboratories we sent samples to didn't care if our clients paid their bills. I was acutely aware that every time I wanted to add a diagnostic test or treatment I had to obtain "approval from the owner." There was no academic department to appeal to if care wasn't approved, no fund of benefactors willing to help owners out. I had to be scrupu-lous.

John had at least ten years on me in the field, and he'd already warned me, "Be careful. You're going to burn yourself out," when I'd eagerly grabbed the phone with a referring vet on the other end. "Burnout" was something I couldn't imagine. To me, more was better. I'd developed a habit of trawling the emergency room in our building for possible cases every day, peering through the cage bars, sneaking a look at treatment sheets, seeing if any of the patients might have a problem I could fix.

I'd found some cases that showed how much I'd learned during my residency. There was the skinny, rumpled, and sad-looking young corgi being treated for unresponsive kidney failure, whose prognosis was worsening by the day. I snagged the record, reviewed the labs, and diagnosed adrenal insufficiency. With some steroids on board, the dog fully recovered and became a long-term patient of mine.

Then there was the tan boxer who barely fit in the cage he occupied. He'd presented with abnormal behavior, due to a profound elevation of his blood sodium level, but no one could figure out why. Ask about his water consumption, I suggested. He hadn't had water for days. His owners had restricted his access to stop him from peeing in the house. We carefully corrected his electrolyte levels and sent him home with more appropriate house-training recommendations. And then there was the case I was called in for to perform an emergency endoscopy. It was a dog who'd, ridiculously, swallowed a cheerleader's baton, somehow cramming the entire thing from his larynx to his stomach. Unfortunately, as much as I wanted to remove the baton with endoscopic prowess, no instrument was large enough to fit through the two-millimeter scope channel and lasso the offending object. I had to relinquish the dog to surgery and go home, but not without first marveling at the X-ray for twenty minutes.

The fire exit slammed when John left the building for lunch. I headed for the treatment room, planning what I'd say to Shannon to advocate for Zeke and his care. I wasn't taking no for an answer this time.

I'd worked myself into a tizzy by the top of the stairs. Already infuriated by the imaginary argument we'd had in my head, I wasn't looking forward to our conversation.

I burst into the treatment room with a falsely cheery smile. "All right. Let's do this."

"Shhh. Be quiet. We're placing Zeke's IV catheter," Shannon replied.

I clenched my back teeth. *Why was it taking so long? Why wasn't he on intravenous fluids yet? Were his blood tests running so I'd have results to help plan my next steps?* The empty tubes lying on the counter suggested this hadn't happened, either.

"Is there anything I can do to help?" I managed.

"No," Shannon replied. "We're good. I guess you could set up the ultrasound if you want."

"I was hoping Zeke would've started fluids by now. I'm worried that he's dehydrated."

"We haven't had a chance. John's ultrasound took longer, and then we had to do aspirates, so we're getting to Zeke now."

"I'm really worried about him. We should've started his treatments by now." I knew it was the wrong thing to say.

"We're getting to it. You're not the only one with patients to take care of." Shannon kept her back to me, carefully taping the catheter into Zeke's vein. He hadn't put up any resistance, another sign of his debilitated condition.

"I understand," I said. "But Zeke's really sick, and his treatments need to get going as soon as possible."

"I know, you've already said that," Shannon replied, hooking up the intravenous fluids hanging on the pole next to Zeke. "How much potassium do you want?"

"Do we have the results of the blood gas yet?" I asked.

"No."

"I was waiting on those results before making a decision about supplementing potassium." I felt her irritation pulse toward me. "I know you'll have to go back and add it later," I said, trying to strike a note of understanding. "But I want to do what's best."

"I do, too," Shannon said, turning to me. "We're still figuring out the way you like things, so you're going to have to be patient."

I heard the accusation in her voice, and I stepped away. This wasn't a battle I'd win. "I'll get the ultrasound set up, then," I said. "Could someone run the coagulation profile to see if I can do a liver aspirate today? Thanks."

I turned away before I could see the reply on Shannon's face.

By the time I'd completed my ultrasound scan, the results of Zeke's blood tests were available. They revealed that Zeke needed a plasma transfusion to replace the clotting factors his liver was unable to make, to reduce the risk of him bleeding uncontrollably from a liver aspiration or feeding tube placement.

Before I could give the transfusion, I had to call Mrs. James to obtain her permission and review the additional cost—carefully choosing my language to imply that Zeke was sick enough to need this extra step, but not that he was too sick to get better. Without placing a feeding tube, I couldn't reverse the damage to his liver. Without a plasma transfusion, I couldn't place the feeding tube.

Mrs. James agreed, and Zeke shuffled a step closer to recovery. He would need an extra night in the hospital before we could safely anesthetize him for feeding tube placement.

The next morning, I arrived early to assess Zeke. I'd made up my mind between midnight and my alarm going off that I was going to place his tube even if his blood-clotting times weren't perfectly normal, and regardless of what Shannon had to say.

I lifted Zeke from his cage and noted that his abdomen was stained a deep yellow from the urine he'd passed overnight. He hadn't the energy to move away, and it had soaked into his skin.

"Morning, Suzy. How's Zeke? He still looks pretty yellow." John had also made it in early.

"He's okay, but his coags were prolonged yesterday, so I was hoping to place his feeding tube this morning. Do you think Shannon could monitor anesthesia and get it going before the day gets too busy?" With John's approval, I knew Shannon would be more willing to help.

"I think so. Let's look at the schedule. As long as Heather can help with appointments we should be fine."

"Thanks. I've been worrying about him all night."

"I know, but you've got to remember that this isn't Penn, and you're used to a different pace. Since you came on board the caseload has increased, and we're all adjusting. We'll probably add more technicians if things stay the way they are, but, for now, try easing off a little."

John's reprimand stung my cheeks, and I remembered the burnout warning he'd given me a few weeks earlier. I wasn't worried about easing off. I was worried about being a disappointment, not practicing well enough, not working hard enough—those were the measures of success I thought everyone valued.

I swallowed my worry and forced neutrality into my voice. "Of course. It's important that the plan works for everyone."

I gently placed Zeke back in the cage, untangling the IV line caught underneath his plump body. He wasn't interested in what I was doing. I wanted him to show me he was okay, maybe with an irritated flick of the paw when I straightened his IV or a swift bat when I opened his mouth to assess his gums, but he remained still.

My procedure was cleared on the schedule, and I prepared the instruments I needed. I caught Shannon appraising me out of the corner of my eye.

"I haven't seen an esophageal tube placed before," she said. "This is going to be a first."

"It's pretty straightforward. It only takes about ten minutes. I like the esophageal placement when I don't want a patient under anesthesia for long."

"John prefers to place gastric tubes. I feel comfortable with those, but for this you're going to have to tell me exactly what you need."

I looked at the materials I'd arranged on the Mayo instrument stand next to the treatment table. I reviewed my mental checklist.

"Do you have a lighter?" I asked.

"What for?" Shannon replied.

"I cut off the end of the catheter at an angle so food doesn't get stuck at the bottom. And then I heat it gently with a lighter so there won't be any sharp edges against the esophageal lining."

"Yeah. I have one." She pulled a lighter from her pocket.

*Interesting,* I thought. *I didn't know she smoked.*

"I think we're ready," I said, reviewing my mental list. "Wait. Let me check one last thing." I scuttled to the opposite side of the room to look at the printout I'd made of the technique the day before. *Right side down, left side up, tube goes in the left side.* It was what I'd thought, but in the final moment I wanted to be sure.

"Is there anything else you need to do before we start?" Shannon asked. "Your first appointment is in thirty minutes."

I kept my back turned to the treatment area and grimaced my answer. My hands were already shaking, and I hadn't picked up the scalpel yet. This would be my first time performing a procedure without the watchful eye of an experienced anesthesia technician and a senior clinician a pager bleep away.

"That's everything," I said. "The sooner we get the tube in, the sooner Zeke will feel better." I kept my tone even and my hands stuffed into the pockets of my white coat until the last minute so Shannon wouldn't notice them quivering.

Despite Shannon's obvious doubts of my ability, once Zeke was anesthetized and she was in control of her patient, the procedure was smooth and uneventful. I showed her how to wrap the tube once I'd placed it, and she agreed to be Zeke's primary caregiver for the remainder of his stay. I was eager to start Zeke's feedings once he'd recovered, to begin reversing the fatty accumulation in his liver, but I had to be patient, gradually increasing his caloric intake over several days until we reached our goal. If he was still doing well at that time, he would go home.

Over the next forty-eight hours we could see Zeke improving. He tolerated his feedings well, and he showed signs that his liver damage was reversing: He began to use the litter box and resumed a more cat-like posture. His lab results confirmed that his bilirubin was decreasing, even though his skin remained alarmingly yellow. His treatments were time-consuming; after the food had been prepared and warmed, it initially took forty-five minutes to administer, so his starved stomach could accommodate the food. Once the process was over, it had to be repeated only a few hours later.

Mrs. James visited daily, and by day four he began responding to her—a clear sign he was going to make it. With his intravenous fluids disconnected, and in an examination room for a visit, he began exploring the environment he was newly interested in. His belly swayed with each meandering step.

"I think he can go home tomorrow," I said when Zeke flopped comfortably onto the floor.

"Are you sure?" Mrs. James asked. "Is he ready? I don't want anything bad to happen at home."

"I think he's ready," I said. "He's feeling much better, and his lab values are all coming down. He's doing very well."

"It's okay if he needs to stay longer. We've talked about it, and we want to do whatever's best."

"I know it seems overwhelming to think about taking him home, but he's going to do just fine."

I watched Mrs. James eye Zeke warily. "I'm not sure about that tube," she said. "I didn't realize it would be sticking out of his neck like that; I'm worried I'm going to hurt him."

"You'll do great. In a few days you'll be a pro!" She couldn't lose her nerve now, not after the thousands of dollars' worth of care Zeke had received. "We'll have everything ready for when you pick him up. Shannon's going to do a feeding with you today as practice. That way it won't seem so scary. I'm going to give you full written instructions, and we'll send home everything you'll need. Can your husband come in as well?"

"I'm not sure if he can get the time off work."

"It would be helpful if he could come. That way I can answer all your questions, and you can both feel comfortable taking Zeke home."

"How long will we need to feed him?" she asked.

"I don't know. Sometimes it's a few weeks, sometimes a month or two. It depends on when Zeke decides to start eating on his own."

"A month or two? That long? You better start eating before that, Zeke, you hear me?"

I smiled. "When the time comes we'll talk about how much Zeke should be eating. It'd be ideal if he could lose some weight. It would be better for his body, and make this less likely to happen again." I looked at Zeke, not wanting to catch his owner's eye.

"I know. We all could, couldn't we, Zeke?"

I laughed unconvincingly, ashamed that I'd transmitted my judgment.

"I'll have Shannon come in to do the feeding with you."

"All right, I suppose we'll give it a shot. What do you say, Zeke?"

I backed out of the room, hoping that Shannon would be her most patient self while going over the feeding instructions.


Zeke made it home, and I monitored him at weekly rechecks. His liver enzymes and bilirubin normalized and his appetite gradually returned, incredibly, with the same gusto he'd had before. I enjoyed Zeke's visits. Each appointment was a step closer to him becoming a normal cat again. His list of medications shrank, and his owner relaxed with each reduction in his treatment plan. I had grown fond of him and his owner. I enjoyed listening to the stories she shared of Zeke before he was sick, and eventually I started hearing stories of his current behavior as he returned to the companion his owner had been scared she'd lose.

At his second-to-last visit, six weeks after his hospitalization, I removed his feeding tube. I snipped through the thick black suture holding it in place and pulled the snake of red rubber catheter through the hole in his skin. I gently cleaned the small puckered mouth of tissue that was all that remained. Once his hair grew back over the area—it was already trying—there would be no lasting evidence of his illness. No lingering abnormalities on serum chemistries, no visible scars, no change in his demeanor. It almost seemed miraculous, except that I understood every step his body had taken back to health.

On his last visit it was time to relinquish his care back to his family veterinarian. Zeke could return to the world of sparse vet visits for vaccinations and teeth cleanings. I was delighted that he'd recovered, but I would miss the familiarity I'd found with his owner over his visits. When Mrs. James left the examination room for the last time with Zeke barely contained in his plastic carrier, she turned and handed me a small package.

"Zeke and I wanted to say thank you," she said.

"Thank you," I replied. "It was my pleasure."

"We've got our old Zeke back," she said. "And we thought we might lose him. Thank you."

I hugged her, trying not to push her off-balance with Zeke dangling in his carrier. I felt a surge of pleasure erasing the arguments with Shannon, my disturbed sleep during his hospitalization, the frustration of not knowing if his owner would proceed. *This is it,* I realized. *This is what it means to be a veterinarian.*

"I was looking through some old photographs the other day," she said, "and wanted you to have this one, to remember Zeke by."

"Thank you. I'm going to put it in pride of place on my desk."

I turned and walked back along the corridor to the double doors that opened into the treatment room. I gripped the rectangular package, reluctant to unwrap it until I knew I'd be alone. I looked at my watch. I had time to sprint downstairs to the office before my next appointment, where I could open the gift and take a moment to compose myself before moving on to the next pet and the next problem.

The picture was taken in a kitchen. It was a candid shot of Zeke caught doing something he shouldn't. A camera grabbed from a drawer when his owner had happened upon him and an open tub of food—busted. A door to a pantry in the background stood half-open. Had Zeke worked at the handle, knowing what was inside, until he figured out the exact amount of pressure to apply? Or had his owner gone to get something and left the door ajar? I liked to think that Zeke was the perpetrator; it fit how I saw him more completely. In the foreground of the picture was a tall, slim Tupperware container; through the clear wall you could see the contents—small brown kibbles. The cat stood on his back legs, his head buried in the container. It was difficult to see his face, but I recognized the closely striped black and silver-brown of Zeke's coat, with its perfectly alternating regularity. His desire to get to the food was both fitting, given the size of his belly, and comic, given his precarious position for his unscheduled snack.

The frigidly bland air of the basement office made me miss, for a moment, the sweltering Philadelphia summer I'd left. It was quiet. There were no pagers bleeping, dogs barking, or monitors alarming. I placed Zeke's picture next to my computer monitor, the first one at my new desk, and clutched my white coat around me. I'd saved Zeke without a senior clinician's advice or an ICU team's monitoring. I grinned thinking of Zeke perpetually captured eating—the very thing that had got him into such trouble. *No wonder he got lipidosis,* I thought, and then stopped myself. *Just enjoy it. Just enjoy this moment.*

# CHAPTER SIX

# Sweetie

I spent two years in Baltimore, achieving board certification and finding my feet as a fully fledged internal medicine specialist. And, although my social circle had shrunk, I was lucky to make the perfect friend to explore my new city with. Robyn was the same age as me, and her exuberant, generous spirit always made me feel I was part of something amazing. She was the head technician for the surgery department of the practice where I worked, and because I never set foot inside the surgical suite, we enjoyed an easy friendship with no work-related conflicts intervening. Robyn was tall with long blond hair, cute dimples, and a personality that made men stare. After three years of veterinarian friendships, it was liberating to not be discussing the most recent *Journal of Veterinary Internal Medicine* article about canine lymphoma on a night out. We spent our weekends shopping, talking, drinking, and chasing boys. It was the most human I'd felt in years.

One Friday in early October 2003, I'd decided on a lazy night in after getting back late from the gym. However, a frantic phone call from Robyn, who'd returned home from work to discover her idiot boyfriend moving his stuff out of their shared apartment, unannounced, instantly changed my plans. We agreed to meet at Kooper's—a bar at walking distance from my apartment, named for the owner's yellow Lab—for sympathy and slander. I'd quickly changed into jeans and my favorite David Gray T-shirt with the provocative lyric IF YOU WANT IT on the front, and COME AND GET IT on the back. I didn't think too much about my outfit; this was going to be a girls' night.

We arrived at Kooper's, grabbed a high-top table against the wall of the bar, and settled in. After gulping down our burgers and pints, we got in a second round of drinks and moved on to lamenting the dearth of smart, interesting, and available men. A speed-dating episode the previous week had failed to supply me with any viable candidates, and I was feeling pessimistic.

"What about these guys?" Robyn asked, nodding toward the entrance of the bar and a group of men, obviously friends, arriving.

"Definite potential," I replied, sliding round to Robyn's side of the table to get a better view. One of them was tall and slim, with a beard a few shades lighter than his thick, dark hair. He wore glasses that were hip before hipsters existed. "That guy with the beard and glasses looks cool."

"Yeah, the blond is cute, too—a bit young, maybe?"

We watched them order drinks, and before I could look away, the guy with the beard and his blond friend approached us.

"We were wondering if you could settle a bet," the bearded guy said.

"Okay," Robyn replied, smiling.

"We're betting on whether or not this jacket is real leather. What do you think?"

I reached for the orange-brown fabric of his seventies-looking jacket and rubbed it. The material was slick and light. "No way," I said. "Definitely not leather."

"Naugahyde, then?" he asked.

"What? You just made that word up. There's no such thing. Nauga—what did you call it?"

We chatted until last call about music, Baltimore, and the things people who've just met in a bar talk about on a Friday night. At closing time, he offered me his business card. *Lame,* I thought, but Robyn and I couldn't stop talking about him on the walk home. Two days later, I was with Robyn and another friend at the annual Fells Point street fair, still talking about the guy from the bar, Rob, when we ran right into him. A chance in thousands.

It was that second meeting that sealed the deal. After I ditched my understanding friends we visited the beer garden, then the Wharf Rat pub, and then a small Egyptian pizza restaurant. He was the man I'd marry. I had no doubt. Rob fit me, and I could see a better version of myself with him around, something no one else had made me feel.

Weekend dates for dinner, drinks, and movies at the indie cinema in town quickly progressed to breakfast at the Blue Moon Cafe the next morning and days exploring Baltimore neighborhoods. "What are you doing tonight?" became "What should we do tonight?" And I figured out exactly how long it took to walk the couple of blocks from Rob's house to my apartment, shower, change, feed the cats, and get to work. When my lease was up at the end of the year we moved into Rob's row home, with only minor adjustments to the décor needed for the four-legged members of the family.

At the hospital, my caseload continued to grow, and even with my new boyfriend waiting at home, I struggled to define the boundary between my work and private life. I persisted in sacrificing dinner plans, social engagements, and sleep for my patients. I was fortunate that Rob was patient and understanding and was self-sufficient enough to not require constant attention.

John, as head of the internal medicine department, continued to warn me that expecting everyone I worked with to share my commitment was unrealistic. The technicians were unhappy, and I was upsetting the balance of the practice. I needed to back off.

But I couldn't do it. No matter the words of warning, or my efforts to "take it easy," when the opportunity to see a case arose, I always grabbed it.

Ultimately, I realized that my philosophy, and that of the people I worked with, was never going to align. I could've looked inward to discover why I couldn't calm my relentless drive, but I wasn't ready. Instead, I chose to move on.

Rob and I moved to San Diego in the summer of 2005. Having lived most of his life in Austin, Texas, Rob was tired of the Baltimore winters, and I'd found what I thought was the perfect practice. He proposed during a Hawaii vacation that summer, and by the following February we were married. But work continued to consume my life, and now I had the full support of a boss whose boundary between work and private life didn't exist.

In contrast to the hospital in Baltimore, my San Diego practice could only be described as old and a bit shabby. The building was barely big enough for the patients, clients, specialists, emergency doctors, interns, and support staff, and the worn floor and scuffed walls showed the strain. A set of thickly painted blue double doors led from the treatment room to a narrow corridor that accessed the six consulting rooms. The constant traffic of people and animals through the doors meant they were a poor barrier between the hospitalization and client areas, and the unpleasant smells generated by sick patients permeated the entire building.

By the end of my first year in San Diego, I was struggling. Despite the long hours I spent in the hospital and the high caseload, I still felt out of place and uncomfortable. In Baltimore, my practice had been the only specialty hospital in the metropolitan area. In San Diego, there were at least four other large emergency and specialty hospitals. Rather than a collegial atmosphere among referral clinics, I'd entered a competition ring. I couldn't say no to any case because, if I did, I'd lose that referring vet's favor. Practicing medicine had become a popularity contest, and I was plunged back into the disorienting social sea of school all over again.

Taking every case meant I had a constantly changing schedule; I had to double-book appointments, and perform unexpected emergency procedures in the middle of the day, which delayed every other patient. My shift didn't finish at a set time; I was done when the last patient was seen and the last record written up. I no longer canceled dinner plans, because I'd learned there was no point in making any.

Though I was spending long hours at the hospital, Rob and I were strengthening our life together. We'd moved into a modern apartment in the central district of Hillcrest. It was a popular and trendy neighborhood, but there was something bland about the bars and restaurants we visited. San Diego was nice—nice weather, nice beaches, and nice people—but it wasn't great. The diversity and texture I'd come to appreciate on the East Coast seemed to have been smoothed away by the surf and sand in sunny SoCal. I missed the tiny Ecuadorean restaurant a block from our Baltimore row home that served the best fried plantains, and our tiny local pub where we knew all the bartenders and they knew what we liked to drink. I missed houses built from bricks, and, when summer changed into fall, most surprisingly, rain. Nevertheless, living in San Diego was fun, and setting up a life with Rob was a shared adventure. I never heard Rob, or the cats—who now had swaths of sunshine to bathe in for days—complain about the new climate.

Although my childhood dreams had always included a pet dog, once I'd adopted my feline family and realized how well-suited they were to my long work hours, I didn't consider dog adoption until Rob became a part of my life. Rob, who was tolerant of the three-cat family he inherited when we met, was not a cat person. The feline behaviors I considered endearing, or at least as part of the package, Rob greeted with less enthusiasm. There were times I felt guilty for my cats' exploits—when Harry vomited in Rob's work shoes or when an anonymous poop appeared in the clothes basket. But my tolerance for cat escapades was significantly higher than my significant other's, and I was sure I had all the pets I needed. However, after Rob had generously put up with the cats for several years and he told me he wanted to add a dog to our family, I couldn't summon valid resistance.

I'd considered myself immune to the homeless dogs I regularly encountered at the hospital. I felt the initial flush of compassion for the individuality, cuteness, or heart-wrenching story of every abandoned, rescued, or abused dog that arrived in our emergency room, but my enthusiasm was quickly cooled by the practical implications of caring for them, and the reality of my long hours.

Professionally, it was prudent to mark the boundaries of my compassion. Internally, I took patients home with me every day. I took records to review at the kitchen table, and I stored lab results in my head to fret over at dinner, in the shower, or in bed at two A.M., but I remained unconvinced that an actual dog would be coming home with me anytime soon. Regardless, dog adoption became a frequent topic during dinner conversation.

Rob erased the lines I'd drawn in the sand, and *nevers* became *maybes*, became *probablys*, became *yeses*. I realized that, for the man I loved, I could tolerate, at least, a four-legged companion of the canine persuasion.

It happened about a year into my new job. I was dodging through the treatment room one day when a patient in the cage closest to the laboratory distracted me. Huddled against the back of the metal cube was a shadow of a dog. Her right hip was up, and the fur was clipped in a neat rectangle framing an incision punctuated by regularly spaced sutures. Her exposed skin looked gray from the black hair follicles crowded beneath the surface. She was quiet, shuttered, separated from the bustle by more than the bars on the door of her cage.

I was drawn to her, forgetting my waiting client. I knelt at the front of the metal cage and looked into her dark brown eyes. She raised her eyebrows in that quizzical, uniquely canine way, but didn't wag her tail or lift her head.

*Who was this dog?* I didn't know anything about her, but I could guess. She was another abandoned pet whose owners couldn't afford her care, dropped at the shelter after being hit by a car. She was a pit bull mix with an injury too severe for medical management, slated for euthanasia because the San Diego Department of Animal Services didn't have the finances for surgery—especially not for a breed already over-represented in their crowded shelter. No one would've argued with the decision to put her to sleep; left to heal on their own, her pelvic fractures would've caused chronic pain and lameness. But someone must have contacted a rescue organization that arranged for her to be taken from the shelter to our hospital for surgery, paid for by fundraising and charitable donations. Someone had saved her life.

I unlatched the cage and sat, the metal floor's sterile coolness on the back of my legs. I could see, now that I was closer, she was not all black; there was a stocking of brindle creeping up each leg, a flash of tigerish stripes on each cheek. Her coat was dull and dusty; when I reached to pet her I felt dirt from the road on her fur. I imagined the smack of the fender, the dull thud of energy absorbed into muscle and bone.

She was unknown, anonymous, defined only by the card on the front of her cage: "Emma." She had no history other than the few words scribbled from the shelter—no likes or dislikes, no favorite toy or special treat. She had no last name, no owner, no home. The cute stories of her as a puppy—I could imagine her as a puppy—were remembered only by those who'd given her up.

Too soon, my technician showed up, hurrying me on to my next appointment. I needed to finish with my client and get on to the next, the constant mantra of the hospital. I reluctantly rose from the cage and patted Emma's head. She subtly shrank from my touch, trying to mold herself to the rigid metal floor. Despite this, when I stepped away she lifted her head slightly as if she missed the pressure of my hand. I looked for the next break in my schedule when I could talk to the surgeon who'd performed her femoral head osteotomy, look at her radiographs to see why the head of her femur had to be removed, and review her bloodwork. My mind was already rearranging the places my three cats occupied, finding more than enough room for a black dog with brindle legs.

Rob and I began by fostering her. But, just like with Monty, I stocked all the necessities. I'd purchased a new brown bed and a matching collar and leash the evening before we took her home. She was discharged a day or two after surgery, with pain medications and instructions to care for her healing bone, muscle, and skin.

I tried to protect myself by thinking of her as Rob's dog, maintaining my boundaries, keeping guard by one fraction of a degree of separation. In truth, there was only a binding and tightening of the bond, not only between Emma and me, but also between Rob and me. As we nursed her back to health, carried her upstairs to bed each night, performed physical therapy exercises for her right hip, and then began short leash walks together, our evolving family solidified. Something had shifted, opened; I'd found that unique place that only a dog could occupy, and Emma fit perfectly.

In those first few weeks we bought her toys and balls, but she wouldn't touch them. She was undoggy in her solitude, making us wonder if something more terrible than a car had hit her. She was too young for such seriousness.

Gradually her leg healed, and her sutures were removed. While her hair grew back she began playing with the toys that had gone untouched for weeks, cautiously chewing on her favorite squeakers until she gained the confidence to rip the small plastic heart out with her strong jaws. And, once she was strong enough, Rob, Emma, and I began to venture out on longer walks together, and then short hikes and, ultimately, visits to Dog Beach. Emma gave us the opportunity to explore parts of San Diego—and our relationship—that we hadn't discovered. She came to work with me and sat in my office while I saw patients. Sometimes I would be gone for hours, rushing between the consulting rooms, treatment room, and procedures area, only returning to the office to grab a file and pick up the contents of the trash can Emma had strewn across the floor in my absence. On the way home I'd call Rob and tell him about her day: the empty food containers she'd licked clean, how she thought anyone who came to the office was there to visit her, the number of times she'd peed and pooped. She was something Rob and I shared in the unforgiving singularity of my work.

About six months after we adopted Emma, I took a case from a referring veterinarian, who, after seeing her patient's pale gums, had requested an emergency internal medicine appointment. Sweetie arrived within the hour.

I could tell by looking across the treatment room that she was a young pit bull terrier, not yet fully grown. Her ears had a soft puppyish flop, her white coat with dove-gray patches looked fresh, and the length of her legs told me she was probably eight or nine months old. She held herself tentatively, lying with her head flat between her front legs and her tail cautiously rubbing the floor whenever someone passed by.

I sat next to her and offered my hand. She raised herself onto her elbows and sniffed my palm.

I carefully petted her head. "Hi, Sweetie, how are you?" I said. But her flash of interest had disappeared and she slumped back onto the hard floor.

Resting my hand on the smooth nape of her neck, I continued talking to her. "I'm sorry you don't feel so good. I'm just going to take a look at you, okay?" I slid my hand along her body and placed my fingers flat against the inside of her thigh. Her pulse felt frantic.

"Good girl. Are you anemic?" I moved back to her head and exam-

ined the color of her gums. I lifted her lip and noted the perfect whiteness of her teeth, confirming her age. Her gums were washed out,
the pink of a drop of blood in a bowl of water. There was a faint
muddy stain on her front legs that suggested she'd been bleeding
from her nose or mouth and had licked away the blood, leaving a
rusty smudge. This explained her weakness and reluctance to stand.

"You are anemic," I said. "How did that happen?" I continued with
my physical examination, palpating her lymph nodes, listening to her
chest. I encouraged her to roll onto her side so I could evaluate the
skin on her belly. The sparse hair there made identifying bruising or
discoloration easier. She flopped more than rolled, and she let out a
soft groan that reminded me of an elderly man lowering himself into
an easy chair. I ran my hand over her abdomen where there were
small, blooming splotches of purple-red blood collected beneath the
skin.

The puce daub over Sweetie's skin and her pale gums suggested
an abnormally low platelet count with severe bleeding as a result. It
was a condition I'd encountered before. I hadn't yet taken a history
from her owners or reviewed the medical record—it was still being
faxed from her regular veterinarian—but I knew what was wrong.
Leaving Sweetie, I lurched on half-asleep legs to the battered central
desk in the treatment room and pulled out a pink treatment sheet
before heading to the exam room.

Sweetie's owners were seated on the short bench opposite the examination table. They were a young couple, huddled together on the
thin blue vinyl cushion. They looked afraid. Their visit to their family
vet to check on blood in Sweetie's urine had turned into an urgent
transfer to a specialty hospital.

The girl took my hand first. She had long, sunny blond hair that
looked like she'd just stepped out of the ocean. She wore sweatpants
designed to look casual and well worn, although the Abercrombie
and Fitch logo told me they were more expensive than the pants I was
wearing. The boy sitting next to her embraced the SoCal skater punk

look, with a corresponding frown. They instantly reminded me of the cool group at school that I'd never been a part of and, despite my white coat and stethoscope, I felt dull and inadequate.

"Hi, I'm the internal medicine specialist taking care of Sweetie," I said, smiling and trying to look professional and reassuring.

"Hi," the girl said. "I'm Stacey. This is Brian." She gestured casually to the boy, and his frown deepened.

"What's wrong with Sweetie?" Stacey asked. "Do you know what's wrong yet?"

"Let's talk about that in a minute," I replied. "First, I want to find out a little more about you and her and what's been going on." My thoughts flicked to Sweetie lying in the treatment room. I was intensely aware that with every minute she was losing more blood.

"Sure." Stacey shifted her weight back and slumped slightly, like a teenager preparing for a parental lecture. Brian remained immobile next to her. They didn't touch or look at each other.

"She was fine until this morning. Last night Brian noticed blood in her urine when she peed on the concrete, but she ate her dinner. This morning, though, she wouldn't get out of bed when we got up, which is super unusual."

"How long have you had Sweetie?" I asked.

"Since she was a puppy. She was about four months old, wasn't she, Brian?" Brian nodded, his gaze fixed somewhere between his knees and the floor.

"A friend's dog had puppies, and Brian had a dog when he was growing up so he wanted to get one. We weren't allowed a dog in our apartment, but when the landlord met her he decided she could stay. That's why she's called Sweetie—she's so sweet."

I smiled at the image of my new patient as a puppy—the perfect pinkness of her newly made foot pads, and the puppyish thump of her paws on the floor of their apartment.

"She must've been so cute," I said. "Has she been spayed?"

We continued through the routine questions. Though I knew that

Sweetie was worsening while I was taking her history, I'd learned that skipping questions and cutting corners would come back to bite me.

"My biggest concern for Sweetie right now is that she's bleeding," I said after I finished taking her history. "I'm worried that she has a dangerously low platelet count which is causing her to bleed uncontrollably." I looked for a sign of comprehension from Stacey, but she stared above my eyeline so intently I wondered if I had a pimple on my forehead I hadn't noticed that morning.

"Platelets are tiny fragments of cells made in the bone marrow," I continued. "They are essential for normal blood clotting, and are constantly plugging up tiny holes in our blood vessels. Without platelets these holes would result in bleeding from everyday activity and normal wear and tear." Sweetie's owners remained impassive. I didn't know whether to interpret their silence as disinterest, or fear.

"Platelets decrease if the bone marrow stops making them or if the immune system destroys them. When the number gets low enough, there is a high risk of severe bleeding from the lining of the nose and mouth, intestinal tract, and urinary bladder. I think that's why Sweetie has blood in her urine. Do you understand so far?"

"I think so," said Stacey. She had shifted forward, resting her elbows on her knees, like she was watching a good TV show. "But what happened to her platelets?"

"That's what we need to figure out. There are many diseases that can cause a low platelet count. There are infections, especially those carried by ticks—"

"I've never seen a tick on her," Stacey interrupted. "Have you, Brian?" She turned to look at him. I caught an inflection of irritation in the question, a hint of accusation.

"Nah, she doesn't go anywhere. She stays in the backyard, and sometimes we take her to Dog Beach." Brian's voice was higher pitched, younger sounding than I expected.

"Ticks aren't common in San Diego," I continued. "But other infections, including those of the urinary tract and skin, can trigger the immune system to eat up platelets like they were a virus or bacteria. Some medications, vaccines, and cancers can also trigger the immune system to destroy platelets. But, honestly, in most cases we never figure out what causes the immune system to turn on itself."

Sweetie had most likely developed immune-mediated thrombocytopenia. Her white blood cells, like microscopic Pac-Men, were gobbling up every platelet in their path, their appetites so voracious that her bone marrow couldn't keep up with demand, and her platelet number had dropped precariously low. Immune-mediated diseases—those that for an unknown or, more precisely, idiopathic, reason resulted in the immune system attacking and destroying the body's own cells—were one of the types of condition I was most interested in.

Rebellious white blood cells didn't have a taste only for platelets. Red blood cells, skin cells, joint cells, and even other types of white blood cells could all come under attack if the immune system was triggered in that specific, peculiar way.

After my second year of veterinary school, I'd taken an extra year to study for a bachelor of science in immunology at King's College. I found the perfect symmetry of an antibody fitting one molecule of an antigen—the cascading dance of cells signaling to and joining one another, the nuanced specificity of one three-letter acronym to another—comforting in its rigor. I had briefly considered a lab-based future, at the forefront of discovery in veterinary immunology, but in clinics I discovered that immune cells were more interesting to me inside bodies than they were in petri dishes.

I liked the wily, fickle, and ruthless nature of an immune system gone rogue. Treating a dog with immune-mediated disease was a battle, and the medications we used to overpower the sophisticated insurgency of a perfectly orchestrated attack were crude, a blanket barrage designed to globally suppress the entire system. Overcoming a rampant immune system was often hard and unpredictable. I'd treated dogs with immune-mediated thrombocytopenia who'd bled uncontrollably and died from blood loss. Others required multiple blood transfusions and immunosuppressive drugs to survive. And some had relapsed one, six, twelve, or even more months later. I didn't yet know which category Sweetie would be in, but I did know that, left untreated, she would be dead within twenty-four hours.

I continued discussing my plan in the exam room with urgency.

"What we need to do now is run some tests to confirm that Sweetie has immune-mediated disease and start treatment. Her age and otherwise good health are on her side, but she may still need to be in the hospital for several days."

"How much is that going to cost?" Stacey asked.

"It's difficult to say. It depends on how Sweetie responds. But it can take three to seven days for the medications to start working, and during that time Sweetie may need multiple blood transfusions. You could easily spend three to four thousand dollars over the next few days."

Stacey looked at Brian and then down at her lap. Brian's position didn't change. They remained separated by a few inches of blue vinyl cushion, but the distance between them seemed greater.

"We don't have that kind of money," she said, not looking up. "Anyway, she was fine last night. I can't believe she's that sick."

"I know it's difficult to understand—how she seemed okay yesterday, and now I'm telling you she needs to be in the ICU," I replied, "but our pets are really bad at letting us know when they're sick, and most of the time we don't realize something's wrong until they're really in trouble. It probably wasn't until Sweetie's platelet count got low enough to cause severe bleeding that she began to feel bad, and that can happen in a matter of hours."

"Why can't we take her home?" Brian asked.

I paused, considering what to say next. The words I used were often alienating in their multisyllabic, clinical nature, and Brian and Stacey had no reason to trust me, other than the authority my white coat suggested. If they took Sweetie home she would almost certainly die. Her gum color and pulse told me she'd already bled to a critical point—she wasn't going to make it without a blood transfusion. Even with a transfusion and ICU care she might not go home. But she wasn't even a year old, and if I could get her through this crisis, she could eventually have a normal life. The medications I'd prescribe to suppress her immune system would likely take a toll over the next four to six months, but in a year or so it might be possible to forget that she'd ever been sick.

More than this, I wanted to save Sweetie for myself. Being the hero felt good, and there was something about Sweetie that reminded me of the moment I met Emma. When I saw the familiar wary need in Sweetie's eyes that day, I thought of the intimate life Rob, Emma, and I shared. The warmth of Emma's body curled next to us on the couch, the smooth velvet of her tongue on the palm of my hand, her doggy, but unique, smell. The particular softness of her ears, and the mumbles, groans, and twitches of her dreams. I wondered if Stacey and Brian felt the same for Sweetie. I tried to imagine their life, how Sweetie greeted them at the door, what they liked to do on the weekend, where Sweetie slept at night.

How strong was the bond that drew these three together? At that moment, in that consulting room, I would put a price tag on Sweetie. It was unpleasant and uncomfortable that this young dog's life depended on how much money her owners were willing—or able—to spend, but it was also reality.

Stacey and Brian faced a common modern dilemma regarding advanced veterinary care—a choice that wasn't available fifty years ago, when veterinary specialties were in their infancy, and the range of medications, surgeries, and treatments for sick pets was restricted to those that could be easily transferred from the large animal world. Today, companion animals occupy a deeper and broader social, economic, and emotional space in our lives than at any time in history.

In 2016, U.S. pet owners spent \$15.95 billion on veterinary care, and that number increases every year. The pursuit of expensive, intensive treatment for our feline and canine companions is a modern choice. And the emotional and financial toll of caring for a sick pet is a luxury afforded to those who choose this road.

Sweetie's owners were young enough to be students, and I won-dered if they'd experienced the illness of a loved one before. I didn't know what I would have done if confronted with the same expense and turmoil when I'd been at vet school.

I brought my thoughts back to the two people sitting opposite me in the exam room. I could see the expanse between myself and Sweetie's owners widening. "Sweetie can't go home," I said. "I know treatment is expensive, but she's critically ill and needs a blood trans-fusion."

"What happens if we don't do that?" Brian asked.

"Bri, we can't take her home. She's going to die if we do, right?" Stacey replied, glancing at him. Brian deflated further into the bench.

"Right. I don't think she'll make it through the next twenty-four hours," I said. "But I understand that it's difficult. It's a lot of money, especially when it's unexpected." I looked at Brian, trying to include him, but he refused to make eye contact.

The room suddenly seemed small and hot. "I'll leave you guys to talk things over while I go and check on Sweetie," I said, half-stepping backward toward the consulting room door. "I'll also have a cost esti-mate made for the next twenty-four hours."

Brian shrugged.

"Okay. Thanks," Stacey replied, looking like she wanted to kick Brian in the shin.

Back in the treatment room, Sweetie was lying where I'd left her. I thought she looked quieter, more withdrawn, but I might've been projecting my anxiety. I found an unoccupied spot at the central doc-tor's desk and cleared a space to finish writing up her treatment sheet. I reviewed the tests and treatment orders I'd planned so far. Sweetie's life-threateningly low platelet count was most likely idiopathic—meaning I wouldn't determine the underlying cause. However, the only way to make that diagnosis was to eliminate all other possibili-ties. This meant performing an array of tests: chest X-rays and ab-dominal ultrasound to look for infections or tumors, bloodwork for tick-borne organisms, a bone marrow aspiration to determine if platelets were being manufactured properly, and serial measurements of platelet count and red blood cell numbers, to decide ongoing treatment.

The first twenty-four hours of testing would likely total over $1,000, not including the cost of hospitalization, intravenous fluids and medications, and, most critically, a blood transfusion, which would easily double the amount. If we were lucky, Sweetie might need only one blood transfusion, and a two-to-three-day stay in the hospital, but there was no way to determine if she would need one or five transfusions, or if her disease would stabilize in a day or two, or a week, or never.

Stacey and Brian had already revealed their financial constraints, and my ideal treatment and diagnostic plans were likely beyond their means. If Sweetie's owners became overwhelmed by the cost, I could lose the opportunity to treat her altogether. Cutting tests and treatments down to the minimum to get us through the next twenty-four hours would make the estimate smaller and less intimidating, but I would run the risk of missing something that could alter Sweetie's outcome. My frustration was familiar and inextricable. What I wanted to do and what I could do for my patient were not the same.

I grabbed a new treatment sheet from the file rack in front of me and threw away the one I'd been working on. I reconsidered my diagnostic plan and began removing tests. My heart accelerated when I imagined the conversation with my new boss. "That's not what I would've done," she would say, and proceed to tell me precisely what she would have done and why, which, I'd determined, rarely lined up with my intended course of action.

For Sweetie, though, what I wanted—more than my boss's approval—was to save her, and I needed to make some decisions before it was too late. I could see Sweetie from my spot at the central desk. Her white flank seemed dazzling in the fluorescent lighting, too clean and bright for the scuffed floor she lay on. I watched the effort she applied to each breath, and noticed the increased rate with which her chest rose and fell, a rapidity that should've been due to playing catch on the beach, rather than her tissues struggling to get enough oxygen because of her declining red cell count. She was too young to die of a potentially treatable disease. I needed to hurry up.

I glanced furtively around the treatment room, looking for the large white-coated frame of my boss, although I would've heard her before seeing her. Her strident voice matched her crimson red lipstick, white-tipped French manicure, and Disney queen black hair. I tried to reassure myself that I knew what I was doing, bolstering my confidence by tallying the patients with idiopathic immune-mediated disease I'd seen, a number so large I couldn't calculate it.

I decided on my course of action and rewrote the treatment sheet. I'd ask the patient advocate—the person formulating and presenting the estimate to Stacey and Brian—to provide two versions of the plan. The first with everything I wanted to do, the second with only the absolute essentials of treatment and monitoring. It was a delicate balance. Often once an owner determined that the cost was too great, their decision became irreversible, no matter the adjustments made. At the same time, if the estimate underrepresented the expense of hospitalization, owners felt duped, angry that costs hadn't been laid out more clearly. But disease was organic and unpredictable, and treatment courses had to be changed and changed again when new problems were discovered—these were factors that were not always possible to account for financially, and not always understandable for those footing the bill. The greatest conflict between my clients and myself in caring for my patients almost always surrounded money.

I got up from the doctor's desk to review my plan with Corey, the patient advocate. I was relieved that she was working the day shift. A small, pretty blonde with a sharp intellect, she had the understanding and empathy to easily make a connection with scared owners and explain treatment plans in a way I couldn't.

"What are they like?" she asked, looking over the treatment sheet.

"They're young, probably your age."

"Wow. I don't have that kind of money." Corey pointed to the four-figure number on her computer screen.

"It's a lot, but have you seen how cute Sweetie is? I think we can fix her, but she needs at least one blood transfusion."

"What's wrong with her?"

"I don't know yet, but I'm guessing immune-mediated thrombocytopenia—the disease where the platelet count gets super low and they start bleeding everywhere."

"Like Patches?" Corey asked, referencing my boss's patient from the month before.

"Yes. But I hope Sweetie doesn't end up like that. Poor dog, I thought her platelets were never going to increase. How many transfusions did she get?"

"Four or five; her owners spent over two thousand dollars just on blood products," Corey said.

"Don't tell Sweetie's owners that," I said.

"Do they have the money?"

"I'm not sure. They're hard to read. I think the girl gets it, but the boy's acting like he doesn't care. If they don't approve the full estimate, I'm hoping we can at least get blood into her and start immunosuppressants. I need you to figure out the most they can spend, so I can figure out what to do."

Corey looked at her computer screen. "We can cut some of the tests?"

"Right," I replied. "I'm hoping we'll get lucky if we treat her for the most common thing."

"I'll see what I can do. Are you going to be here or in your office?"

"Here," I said, feeling the need to stand vigil over my new patient while her fate was decided. "Good luck."

Corey got up from her desk and pushed through the double doors leading to the consulting rooms. All I could do was wait.

Corey returned to the treatment room fifteen minutes later.

"So?" I asked.

"I don't know yet. They don't have the money. I gave them the CareCredit stuff, but they probably won't qualify because they're students. Stacey's calling her dad to see if he'll help out. If not, I don't think they can even afford the CBC."

I looked at Sweetie and thought of Emma. "Maybe I could take her," I said. "Maybe Emma needs a playmate."

"Are you kidding?" Corey asked.

"I don't know," I replied. Imagining Emma and Sweetie curled on the couch, romping on the beach, walking on matching leashes. "She really reminds me of Emma, and if I don't treat her, she'll die."

Every day I encountered financial constraints—canceling diagnostics and omitting treatments. I'd euthanized patients due to the cost of necessary care and the lack of reasonable alternatives. If Sweetie's owners declined the estimate, I had three choices: First, send her home with my best guess at treatment and hope she didn't die from blood loss overnight. Second, I could assume her ownership and the associated treatment costs. Or third, I could put her to sleep, knowing that without a blood transfusion it was unlikely that she'd make it, and to send her home would only prolong her suffering.

It wasn't completely unprecedented for me to consider adopting Sweetie, but it was a scenario that hospital management tried to avoid—sometimes the original owner would have a change of heart and demand their pet be returned, or the staff member trying to do the right thing could be left with an unexpectedly large bill for which they were no more equipped to pay than the original owner.

In most cases, animals were saved from euthanasia by the same complicated emotional connection I felt the first time I met Emma. A first-date kind of instinct that this pet was the right one—likely based on the same multitude of factors that determine the people we choose to surround ourselves with. In some cases, though, more pragmatic reasoning would result in an animal being saved. Young cats with urinary tract obstructions, like Tiger, who needed vital care but could fully recover, were occasionally adopted into the hospital's feline blood donor program if their temperament was good and the only other option was euthanasia. After screening for the blood-borne infectious diseases feline leukemia virus, feline immunodeficiency virus, and the red blood cell parasite *Mycoplasma haemofelis,* suitable cats would join the small colony of three to four others that lived at the hospital to provide blood for transfusion to critical feline patients.

Cat blood was difficult to collect and store, making on-site donors the best option for supplying whole blood for transfusion to bleeding or anemic patients. By 2007, when I met Sweetie, canine blood banking in the United States was well established, but the technology for separating and storing feline blood components was still in its infancy.

The first commercial U.S. canine blood banks were established in the late 1980s. Donor dogs, often from rescue organizations or specific breeding facilities, are screened for infectious diseases, temperament, and blood type, and then owned and housed by the blood bank. Animal Blood Resources International, the first commercial pet blood bank, reports that they rehome their in-house blood donors after one year of service. Hemopet, the first nonprofit animal blood bank, established in California in 1986, houses a closed colony of rescued greyhounds. They donate blood on average twice a month for twelve to eighteen months, and are then rehomed. These retired racing dogs seem like ideal blood donors, with their known medical history, docile personality, and perfect anatomy—prominent veins, a thin hair coat, and lean body condition.

Since animal blood banks first became available, alternative methods for obtaining donors have become increasingly popular, given the potential animal welfare concerns about housing dogs solely for blood donation. Volunteer canine blood donation programs are now well established by universities and charitable organizations across the United States. Typically, healthy dogs over fifty pounds, between one and five years of age, and who test negative for blood-borne infectious disease, are eligible to become volunteer donors. Owners may bring their dogs to a set location, or mobile blood banks travel to communities to increase the accessible donor pool. The University of Pennsylvania's Penn Vet Bloodmobile has pioneered this approach. Volunteer dogs are rewarded with a biscuit, a bandanna, and a belly rub. Their owners enjoy the knowledge that they are helping save other dogs' lives, and both dogs and owners seem happy with the deal.

In the late 1990s, when I was in vet school, British animal welfare laws dictated that blood could be drawn only from a live donor and given immediately to the recipient. The storage, or banking, of animal blood products was illegal. I understood the concerns of the British government—that for-profit blood-banking services might sacrifice animals for financial gain. Donor dogs exsanguinated to obtain blood products, and live donors kept in poor conditions to maximize the profit from their moneymaking donations, were practices whispered about in the United States. How, after all, did a dog provide consent for its donation of 450 milliliters of blood?

It wasn't until October 2005, after my arrival in San Diego, that British legislation permitted the banking of canine blood products by nonprofit organizations for transport to other veterinary facilities. By that time, I thought little about the ethical implications of using banked blood products; they were a standard part of my care for any animal that needed them.

The feline donors in San Diego were typically those rescued from euthanasia for fixable problems. They led a decent life in a cat tree–adorned run in a quiet area of the hospital. They donated blood every sixty to ninety days, but I was guilty of flouting the rules when I had a critical patient in need of a transfusion and no donors were available. Sometimes the ethical considerations of feline blood donation tripped me up.

Were we exploiting our donor cats for the sake of more-loved pets?

It was a question I didn't consider when ordering blood for my canine patients, but I thought more carefully when it came to cats. More recently the storage and separation of feline blood has become feasible, and blood banks now house colonies of cats to supply demand and, ultimately, be adopted out. But the long-term consequences of repeated sedation and blood donation can include renal failure, iron deficiency, and cardiac failure. These are risks that canine blood donors, due to their large size and ability to donate without sedation, do not run.

Similar to humans, dogs and cats have specific blood types, with similarly serious consequences if incompatible blood is transfused. Cats, like humans, have naturally occurring antibodies to red blood cells of a different type, while dogs do not form antibodies to DEA (dog erythrocyte antigen) until they've been exposed to blood products. Blood-borne infectious disease screening, typing, and cross matching are necessary requirements in veterinary transfusion medicine, as they are in humans.

I considered my options for Sweetie. She hadn't received previous blood products, and I was willing to administer a red cell transfusion without a cross match. But I didn't yet know if I'd be given the chance to try.


I resumed my position on the floor next to Sweetie while Corey and I waited for her owners' decision. I anticipated the flurry of technicians, catheters, and blood tubes once the estimate was agreed upon. I tested the idea of adopting Sweetie if her owners declined treatment, forming the picture of adding another dog to our family, prodding our routine gently like a Jenga tower to see if it would fall down. I would need to speak to Rob, and I could predict his practical answer, removed from the emotion of the treatment room. We didn't have space for another dog in our lives.

A receptionist popped her head round the treatment room door.

"Corey, they're ready for you again in five."

"Let me know if you need me," I said when Corey passed by on her way to the exam room.

Corey didn't take long. "They want to talk to you," she said. "Well, Stacey does; Brian's outside smoking. It sounds like her dad might be up for lending her some money."

"Okay, wish me luck," I said.

In the consulting room Stacey seemed younger than she had fifteen minutes earlier. She was alone, and had pulled her feet onto the bench, hugging her knees. She seemed incapable of making a decision about what to eat for lunch, much less about whether to approve treatment for her dog.

"Brian's outside," she said after I'd closed the door. "He's freaking out about Sweetie. He really loves her."

"That's okay. I'm sure everything seems overwhelming right now, and everyone handles stress differently."

Stacey shrugged. I wondered how much longer Brian would be around.

"I spoke to my dad," she continued. "He's out of town, but he said he'd lend me the money. He always visits Sweetie when he's around. Sometimes I think he likes her more than he likes me. He'll lend me eight hundred, and I can get two hundred in the next day or so. There are some people who owe me money. Do you think that's enough?"

Stacey looked at me in a way I imagined she looked at Brian, or her dad, when she wanted something.

*A thousand dollars.* A thousand dollars wasn't much when it came to a dog in need of a blood transfusion and a hospital stay. "If Sweetie only needs one transfusion and we can get her home in a day or so I think we'll be okay. I'm going to cut most of the tests to use the money for treatment," I said.

"Is she going to make it?"

I paused. I didn't know the answer. "I hope so," I replied. "Most dogs with her condition do well with treatment, but occasionally, even with all the money in the world, we can't save them."

"We could spend all this and Sweetie not come home?" Stacey frowned. "My dad'd kill me if she dies now."

"I wouldn't recommend treating her if I didn't think she had a good chance. But medicine isn't exact, and we don't know what's going to happen until we try."

"We should treat her, then?"

"Absolutely. I think we can get her through this."

"Okay, I guess. What do I do now? Can I see her?"

"I'll have Corey go over the paperwork and then we'll bring you back to see her."

I stepped out of the room and rearranged Sweetie's plan in my head, tallying tests into *essential, maybe,* and *not necessary* columns on an imaginary worksheet. I walked back to Corey's desk, considering how best to spend a thousand dollars.

"What's the deal?" Corey asked.

"We have a thousand dollars. Most from her dad, and the rest she's going to make up somehow."

"A thousand?" Corey looked skeptical. "The original estimate was for three."

"I know, but it's all we've got. Let's start again."

Corey pulled up a blank form on the monitor. I named a test or treatment, she typed it in, and we watched the number in the top right corner of the screen climb. We had enough funds for one night of hospitalization, routine bloodwork, a set of X-rays, and, most important, one blood transfusion.

I thought about what a blood transfusion would provide. Sweetie's main problem was a lack of platelets—which would not be replaced by a packed red blood cell transfusion. The best we could hope for was that the transfusion would buy us time while we waited and hoped for the immunosuppressants to kick in. Platelets are delicate, microscopic fragments of cells that are irretrievably damaged by the process of blood collection and storage—like fragile spring flowers that wilt and lose their color the moment they are plucked from the ground. Even if platelet-rich plasma, a costly and highly specific blood product, were available to replace her platelets, her overactive immune response would eat them as quickly as they could be poured in.

One unit of packed red blood cells would consume almost five hundred dollars, and until her platelet count increased Sweetie could continue to bleed excessively. One unit of blood could be a drop in the ocean. But what other options did I have?

*There was one,* I realized.

"Do we have any empty collection bags?" I asked Corey.

"You'd have to check with Sylvia, but I think there are usually one or two in the hospital."

"Thanks," I replied. I'd been asking myself what I'd do if Sweetie were my dog, since the thought of scooping her into my family first crossed my mind. I considered the slick, dense bag of packed red cells sitting in the refrigerator. We had one chance, and I doubted that a single bag was enough. But if I could find a donor to give a unit of fresh whole blood, I could deliver it immediately to Sweetie. It was likely that the extra clotting factors, the tiny number of functional platelets, and the fresh red cells would do more good than a unit of older, dying, red blood cells. Whole-blood donations were typically separated into cells and plasma to most fully utilize the components. With an on-site donor, maybe a young, healthy pit bull mix with a black coat and brindle legs, I could give a unit of fresh whole blood that was greater than the sum of its parts.

Emma was sitting in my office. She was healthy and young; she was the right weight—the perfect donor. She and I could be heroes. I imagined an extra life-giving force infused with Emma's blood into Sweetie's veins once the transfusion began.

That Emma was still nervous to the point of distress in unfamiliar situations, and that she cowered and hid at the sight of certain members of the hospital staff, didn't deter me from granting her consent.

*Would Rob agree to Emma being a blood donor?* I considered calling him, but it was the middle of the day, and he was probably busy. I didn't have time to talk everything through with him. And ultimately, if he said no, I knew I wouldn't abide by his decision. The needs of my patient were more pressing than Emma's potential distress or my husband's consent. I wanted to save Sweetie, and, if I gave her Emma's blood, I could quantify her improvement by checking her bloodwork, feeling her pulse, and examining the color of her gums. There was no way to document Emma's reaction in such a reassuring way. Even if Emma's distress at being lifted onto a table and restrained on her side for twenty minutes—while her blood flowed from a large needle placed in her jugular vein, through transparent plastic tubing and into the collection bag—became too great, I was willing to give her sedation to obtain the lifesaving fluid if I needed to.

*The greater good,* I told myself. Emma's blink of discomfort could save Sweetie's life. For me, it was an easy decision.

Emma was reluctant to be led into the treatment room. The last time she'd been there, I realized, was the day we'd taken her home. At the treatment door, she lowered her head and braced her legs, as if the doorway was a cliff edge I was asking her to jump from.

I tugged gently at her leash. "Come on, Emma, it's going to be okay," I said.

We first needed to check Emma's blood type and red blood cell count, and run a quick infectious disease screen, even though her chances of having contracted a transmissible disease were low, given her reluctance to do anything much more than lie on our couch. Sweetie also needed to be set up—have blood drawn, an intravenous catheter placed, and IV fluids started. And I had another patient waiting to be seen.

Emma was a compatible donor, and Sweetie's bloodwork confirmed that she needed a blood transfusion. Among appointments, checking on Sweetie, and the hustle of a regular workday, I tried to remain solicitous of Emma's care. I'd entrusted her to Nicole, the head technician on the internal medicine service. Nicole was tall, slim, and blond in a way that could have been attractive but instead was angular and awkward. Her poorly veiled displeasure directed at me—the new doctor, trained on the East Coast, who didn't do things the way they should be done, or, at least, not the way "the boss would do them"—made me miss cranky but straightforward Shannon from Baltimore.

I'd become familiar with Nicole's running commentary of "Are you sure?," "I haven't done it that way before," and "Why don't you check with the boss?" whenever I asked for a particular test or treatment to be performed in a specific way. Her constant doubt leached into the other technicians on the service, forming a divide that wasn't easy to overcome. Despite this, I knew that Nicole was experienced and competent, and that she'd get the job done.

"Emma needs sedation," she told me on one of my visits to the treatment room between appointments.

"Really?" I looked at Emma, who seemed to be suctioned to the floor, quivering as if she'd lost control of voluntary muscle movement. "What happened?"

"She won't sit still, and I don't have time to wrestle with her."

"Have you tried less restraint? She's really nervous. She might do better with that."

Nicole looked at me like she'd smelled something terrible. "She needs sedation," she replied curtly.

I hadn't seriously considered sedation or Emma's quivering fear when I'd thought up my brilliant, lifesaving plan.

"How about if I try holding her?" I asked, glancing at the clock and realizing that I didn't have time to do anything other than see my next patient.

"You'll probably make things worse," Nicole replied. "Just write up the drugs you want so we can get this blood." She turned away from me before I could respond. I located Emma's treatment sheet to write up her sedation. It was a standard drug combination that I used on many patients when they were too nervous, uncomfortable, or wiggly to allow routine testing such as X-rays and ultrasound. But, even with the safest drugs, sedation could sometimes cause unexpected side effects, and there was always the risk of cardiovascular compromise. For a young, healthy dog like Emma, sedation was unlikely to cause a problem, but the thought of giving her drugs she didn't need for a procedure that wasn't going to help her was unpleasant and nerve-racking. *Shit, what have I done?* I thought. *What if Emma had a reaction to the sedation or didn't recover well?* It was too late to back out. I turned away, not trusting the color rising to my cheeks.

"Be gentle with her," I said, heading out of the treatment room.

Nicole didn't reply.


"Sweetie is stable," I said to Stacey on the phone later that day. "She's tolerating her blood transfusion well."

"What did her tests show?"

"Her bloodwork confirms what we suspected—her platelet count is very low, and she's very anemic."

"She has that thing you talked about? What's it called?"

"Immune-mediated thrombocytopenia—her immune system is eating up her platelets."

"Is she going to die? You said some dogs die from that disease, right?"

"We have to see how she does after the transfusion. She's stable right now, and hopefully she'll feel better with more red blood cells."

"I feel so bad. It's my fault if she dies," Stacey said. I heard stifled sobbing coming from the phone. "Brian says we can't spend any more money, and we have to take her home tomorrow, no matter what." She hiccupped the last word.

"It's not even his money," she continued. "But Brian says if we spend everything on Sweetie there won't be enough left for the wedding." She sniffed. "Can't you help us out? I'd do anything to save her. I'd pay off her care, or you could give me a discount. I'm a student."

"Unfortunately, I don't control the cost of Sweetie's care. You can talk to Corey about the bill next time you speak." I didn't want to bargain over Sweetie's life.

"You're doing everything you can," I said. "We're giving Sweetie the best care, and so far there's no indication that she's not going to make it."

I thought about telling her that Sweetie was receiving my own dog's blood. That I meant it when I said we were doing everything possible. That I was already feeling remorse for my decision to help Stacey's dog without regard for my own, for not telling Rob about what I'd done. But I decided against it. The whole thing was too personal to share with someone I didn't know. I hung up, after promising updates if Sweetie worsened overnight, and a call in the morning once I'd assessed her. Before I'd called Stacey, I'd gently ushered Emma back to the office to continue recovering. She was still heavily sedated, and lay sprawled on the office floor. I hoped she'd wake up before it was time to leave.

When Emma and I got home that night she was still disoriented and agitated. I had to help her out of the car under Rob's quietly displeased gaze. My reasonable explanation for sedating our dog and taking her blood, without discussion, sounded dry and hollow when I gave it to Rob. In the hospital, Emma's role in Sweetie's care was barely acknowledged. In the veterinary world, it was ordinary, if not expected, that our personal pets would be a part of the treatment plan if required. Our list of blood donors extended to those healthy dogs and cats of the right age and weight owned by hospital employees.

But the parameters of normal I was used to in the clinic didn't extend beyond its automatic doors. Jokes about anal sac expression, and the gallows humor of caring for sick, dying animals every day, didn't translate to after-work drinks banter with anyone other than vets. But Rob wasn't a vet, and no matter how tolerant he was of the long hours, intrusive phone calls, canceled plans, and my growing list of work-related frustrations, I'd never before crossed the line between work and home so completely. I had stepped away from the implicit compact of our relationship by excluding him from a decision about Emma that, now that we were a family, he should've been a part of. I realized that he would've consented to Emma giving blood if I'd asked, would've trusted my judgment that I was making a choice that was reasonable and safe, but I hadn't asked. I had chosen to pursue the course that best suited me, and the payoff for doing so, I recognized, was small.

Rob's annoyance was mild and short-lived, but my guilt was slower to fade, and Emma's sedation didn't fully wear off until the next morning. By then I was exhausted from a night interrupted by Emma's confused and disoriented pacing and whining, and my own remorse.

When I arrived at the hospital, Sweetie looked better. It was too early to expect her bruising to be fading, but she wagged her tail more vigorously when she saw me. Her gums, though still pale, were turning pink, and her heart rate had slowed, suggesting she was holding on to the red blood cells she'd received.

Her test results confirmed that her anemia had improved, and she ate a little breakfast—a good indicator she was feeling better. I'd started immunosuppressive steroids the day before, but one dose couldn't have influenced her platelet count yet. She wasn't out of the woods. Until her platelet count increased she could bleed uncontrollably, and possibly fatally, at any time. I wanted Sweetie to stay in the hospital several more days, until her risk of bleeding diminished, but Stacey and Brian's one thousand dollars would be gone by early evening, and Sweetie would be going home.

I worried that what I'd put Emma through might not be enough to save Sweetie. I couldn't control what would happen to her once she was out of the hospital. I could only give her owners discharge instructions and pill bottles. Whether Stacey remembered that Sweetie shouldn't eat hard food or chew on toys until her platelet count was normal was out of my hands. I imagined Sweetie dying in the backyard, bleeding into the ground while Stacey was at class. I expected her to show up in the emergency room weak and lethargic, in need of another blood transfusion. And I thought, for a moment, about how she could've become my pet, and how, in that scenario, I'd be charged with the months of medications and monitoring I was entrusting to Stacey and Brian. An evanescent sadness left me with the relief that I wasn't going to be the one to get up every two hours to take Sweetie outside to pee—a common side effect of steroids.

"Call me if you have any questions," I said, standing in the same exam room I'd met Stacey and Brian in only a little over twenty-four hours earlier. Stacey was alone. I didn't ask where Brian was, but I wondered if they wouldn't need the money for a wedding after all.

"And remember that the emergency room is always open, so if you're worried you can bring her in anytime."

"Do you think she'll be okay?" Stacey asked.

"If we can get her through the next few days and her platelet count comes up, then I think she'll make a full recovery," I replied, sidestepping the question.

"I know you think we should be keeping her here longer, but she'll be happier at home." Stacey looked away. I imagined the conversation between her and Brian before she'd arrived at the hospital, convincing themselves that the reason they were bringing Sweetie home was that it was in her best interest.

She had put herself in a tough position to save her dog. It was possible that the eight hundred dollars Stacey now owed her father would cause lingering arguments and resentment, and the money she and Brian had pitched in might mean they wouldn't make that month's rent. Was it going to be worth the sacrifice if Sweetie didn't pull through?

It was hard to accept that the rest of Sweetie's recovery was beyond my influence. I couldn't control her owners' financial situation, and I couldn't affect the choices they would make now that Sweetie was out of the hospital. It was hard watching her and Stacey leave that night, not knowing if I'd see Sweetie—who now carried something of Emma inside her—again. I'd scheduled Sweetie for a recheck in forty-eight hours—her platelet count would either be increasing or she'd need another blood transfusion by then. *If she isn't dead*, I thought grimly.

Two days later I waited impatiently for Sweetie to arrive for her recheck. I'd called Stacey the day before to check on them, but I'd only got a voicemail message. Did that mean Sweetie wasn't doing well? Or was she doing better? Or was she dead? I tumbled the possibility over and over until she showed up in my exam room at her appointed time.

My relief at seeing Sweetie was matched by her exuberant doggy greeting—all tail wag, pink tongue, and wiggling. She looked good. Her gums were pink and the bruising on her belly had faded to the mottled purple-yellow of a ripe Victoria plum. I felt confident that her platelet count would be in the normal range on her bloodwork. In my mind, Emma's blood was rushing through Sweetie's body vanquishing the rogue white blood cells. I was sure that Emma had given more to Sweetie than a mix of red and white cells; a few platelets; and the fluid, proteins, and other molecules of plasma. It was the same archaic belief the first physicians performing blood transfusions in the seventeenth century firmly adhered to: that the essence, or character, of the donor could be transferred to the recipient through blood.

The results of Sweetie's CBC showed that her platelet count had increased to 70,000, lower than the 200,000 considered normal but out of the danger zone. I predicted that it would continue to rise and that her bruises would fade over the next few days.

Stacey and Sweetie returned again a week later. Sweetie's platelet count had returned to normal—she'd survived the critical period. I warned Stacey that it was too early to alter her steroid dosage, but that if all went well, we would taper, and discontinue, the medication over the next four to six months. I warned her that Sweetie could relapse if medications were weaned too quickly, or if regular monitoring was missed. But I could already see the distance and complacency of invincible youth in Stacey's eyes. The danger had passed, and Stacey was already remembering Sweetie's illness differently. When she reluctantly agreed to bring Sweetie back in a month I wasn't sure she'd keep the appointment. I considered, then, telling her the story of Emma. But it was too late. Sweetie was well. My revelation might garner a shrug or muttered thanks, but it wouldn't guarantee that I'd see either of them again.

After that visit Stacey would initially answer my phone calls and promise to bring Sweetie in, but they never appeared on my schedule.

I'd saved Sweetie, using my knowledge and experience to treat her within her owners' economic constraints. But the victory seemed slight. I'd crossed the line between my professional and private lives, and I'd drawn Emma into the battle without consideration of her welfare, or my husband's consent. The edges of internal medicine had smoothed like a pebble tumbled by the tide of my patients, but I was still struggling to find the balance between my career and myself.

CHAPTER SEVEN

# Grayling

D r. and Mrs. Dixon perched like hedgerow birds on chairs
pushed against the wall of my consulting room. Their feet
dangled childishly a few inches from the floor, and I loomed above
them. Their dog, Grayling, was a six-year-old, 140-pound Irish wolfhound who'd been transferred into my care that morning from the
emergency room. Each member of the small, older couple weighed
significantly less than their choice of canine companion. I was intrigued.

I was struggling to treat Grayling for an unknown but aggressive
infection. She'd come into the hospital the previous afternoon with a
fever, high heart rate, and reluctance to walk—I couldn't help wondering how her owners had transported her. Although her physical
examination and bloodwork had suggested a life-threatening bacterial infection—sepsis—her chest X-rays and abdominal ultrasound
had failed to reveal the source of the infection, and she'd continued to
decline overnight despite intravenous fluid and antibiotic therapy.

The hospital grapevine had already informed me that Dr. Dixon

was a retired pediatric neurologist and his wife, a retired nurse. I suspected his attire of a gray tweed suit, with a hunter green pocket
square, shirt, and tie, was similar to the outfit he'd worn each day to
clinics before his retirement. Maybe back then, a reflex hammer
poked from his jacket pocket or a stethoscope hung from his neck.
Despite his sparse white hair and lightly angled posture, his eyes were
vibrant. His wife's hair was gray and closely cropped. She wore sensible brown shoes, a pair of what my grandmother called "slacks" in
a comfortable, practical fabric, and a light sweater in a shade of
mauve favored by those over sixty.

I expected that when they answered my questions they would
speak with a Scots-Irish brogue. Dr. Dixon's suit seemed more appropriate for the Scottish Highlands than a San Diego beach, and I imagined that the breed heritage of their dogs—two Irish wolfhounds and
a Scottish deerhound—would be reflected in their nationality. I was
slightly disappointed, then, when they spoke in well-clipped American, East Coast accents, reminiscent of a PBS history show.

Grayling was already occupying the floor next to the first large
cage by the treatment room door—due not only to her gargantuan
size but also the severity of her condition. Irish wolfhounds were
relatively rare patients in San Diego. My typical canine population
was tipped in favor of smaller breeds—Chihuahuas, various sizes and
shapes of terrier, and a seemingly infinite variety of small, white,
fluffy dogs. Then came the Labrador and golden retrievers, numer-
ous iterations on the theme of pit bull terrier, and a smattering of
dachshunds, schnauzers, pugs, boxers, and other breeds (or non-
breeds) that ranged in weight from one to greater than 180 pounds.

The difficulties of caring for a 140-pound dog weren't limited to
finding an adequately sized cage. From performing a physical examination to calculating the volume of antibiotics to administer, everything had to be super-sized for Grayling. That morning I'd encountered
a recumbent dog who weighed more than I did. She was too weak to
stand, which made performing a thorough physical examination to
identify a possible source of infection surprisingly difficult.

Grayling lay on her side, and I sat on the floor next to her. She lifted her head an inch or so off the ground to acknowledge my presence, but then failed to respond to me further. Her coat was a light, silvery gray with the faintest sandy brown hair behind her ears, under her chin, and on her upper legs, and although it looked coarse and wiry, it was soft. She was a little overweight, likely a reflection of her San Diego lifestyle, where her daily exercise consisted of neighborhood walks, rather than the hunting and tracking in the Highlands she'd been designed for. I noticed that Grayling's right legs were slightly swollen when compared to her left. This suggested that she'd been lying on her right side too long, despite the technicians' efforts to keep her propped on her chest. I added two-hourly adjustments of her body position to her treatment sheet to prevent pressure sores, and dependent edema—fluid accumulation under the skin—from developing.

I began at her head, methodically working through the order of physical examination I'd performed thousands of times before. I was not only assessing her overall status, but was also looking for clues to how an infection had entered her body. I looked carefully in her mouth for signs of a tooth root abscess or areas where a piece of stick or other foreign material might have penetrated her oral mucosa. I palpated her peripheral lymph nodes, feeling for asymmetry or changes in shape, size, or texture that might hint at an initial site of infection. I auscultated her chest, listening for subtle signs of fluid in her lungs, but I couldn't assess her right side. It was impossible for me to lift her chest high enough to slide my stethoscope between her and the vinyl-covered foam mat she lay on. Her abdominal palpation also proved challenging. Effectively palpating Grayling's abdomen would have required her to stand so I could use both hands to feel for the margin of her liver, spleen, kidneys, and bladder, while also assessing for thickening, enlargements, or masses. But getting Grayling to stand was impossible, and even if I'd achieved this feat, discerning individual organ margins in her massive abdominal cavity would've been difficult. I knew I might miss important clues.

Sitting on the corner of the mat, I reviewed my findings. The physical examination had divulged little, other than my preference for patients I could pick up, so I turned my attention to other possible causes of her condition—a penetrating wound, a venomous spider or snake bite, or an infection originating in her intestinal tract that had leaked into her circulation. I combed my fingers through Grayling's thick, silvery coat. The hair on her legs was dense, designed for tracking wolves through thick undergrowth. The bite of the black and brown widow spiders and the rattlesnakes that were native to San Diego could leave almost invisible puncture marks. Two tiny, perfectly spaced spots may be the only evidence, sometimes not apparent until a day or two later when the toxins injected under the skin caused necrosis and severe inflammation. Unless I knew exactly where she'd been bitten it was unlikely I'd find the punctures, if they existed.

I ran my hands down her legs, feeling for swelling or heat around her joints, parting her hair to look for reddening or bruising of her skin. She felt hot all over; her last recorded body temperature was significantly elevated, but it was hard to determine any heat differential through her coat. I considered finding help to encourage Grayling to stand while I evaluated her lungs and abdomen more fully. But the slick, easy-to-clean hospital flooring was a challenging surface for weak dogs with unsteady legs and slippery paws.

Grayling's quiet demeanor was likely a combination of the severity of her illness and her natural disposition. A calm, stoic personality was a constant among the few Irish wolfhounds I'd cared for. They seemed most content lying on the exam room floor, nose between their outstretched legs, paying little attention to what was going on around them. Grayling's owners indicated that she was of a similar nature, happiest when she was lying on the couch—I wondered if they perched, one on each arm of the sofa, or if they were forced to sit on the floor.

The thought of Grayling and her two humongous canine housemates living with Rob and me jumped into my head. I couldn't picture even one of them joining us. We didn't have the room or the time for the amount of hair they'd shed, food they'd eat, bowel movements they'd produce, and dirt they'd carry in on their paws. Patients like Grayling made me grateful that Emma could reasonably join me, Rob, and our three cats on our couch.

After performing Grayling's physical exam, I shifted my attention to her owners. Dr. and Mrs. Dixon were deliberate and thoughtful in their answers to the questions I posed, with a synchronicity between them that was the result, I assumed, of a long and happy marriage. My history-taking, in contrast, felt urgent. I was desperate to determine the source of Grayling's infection and improve our chances of effectively treating her given her poor response to antibiotic therapy over the previous twelve hours.

"Has Grayling traveled outside San Diego?" I asked.

"Oh yes, we take her and her brothers to Canada every summer," said Mrs. Dixon.

"You do? How do you get there?"

"We drive," Mrs. Dixon replied.

"All the way?"

"Well, yes. How else would we do it?" Dr. Dixon replied, smiling at his wife in response to my poorly veiled surprise. "We go in the minivan. A few days there, and a few back. We share the driving all the way to Vancouver. The dogs love the trip."

I pictured a minivan crammed with three large dogs and all their accoutrements as well as Dr. and Mrs. Dixon. I stifled the many questions I wanted to ask and instead returned to the relevant ones. "When was the last time you were there?"

"Last summer," said Dr. Dixon. "We usually go from June to the end of August. We were planning on leaving in a few weeks, but now we might have to wait for Grayling."

"Has she had any previous medical problems?" I continued.

"Not really," Mrs. Dixon replied. She looked at her husband for confirmation.

"She had diarrhea last summer," Dr. Dixon said. "They all did. The vet in Canada said it was giardia, most likely from the deer poop they were eating."

A clue? But it was too long ago to be causing her current, acute problem.

"She hasn't had diarrhea since?" I asked.

"No," said Dr. Dixon, his wife concurring with a nod. "Everything was fine until yesterday morning, when she was suddenly not herself. By lunchtime she looked worse, and we decided to bring her to the emergency room."

"And nothing's changed recently? Could she have been bitten by a snake or spider?"

"I don't think so," said Mrs. Dixon. "We tend to just walk around the neighborhood in San Diego. The dogs prefer hiking in Canada, don't they, dear?"

"That's right," Dr. Dixon said. "There's been no change from our routine."

I'd exhausted my questions, and I was no closer to solving the mystery.

"What we know so far is that Grayling most likely has an overwhelming bacterial infection causing sepsis," I said. "But we don't know where it's coming from. We haven't found pneumonia or a kidney or bladder infection, and I haven't identified any wounds that could be seeding her blood with bacteria."

"Could it be a viral infection? A viral meningitis, say?" asked Dr. Dixon, reminding me of his background in pediatric neurology.

"It's possible," I replied. "But viral infections in dogs are relatively uncommon. The only viral meningitis we see is caused by distemper, which is unlikely given Grayling's age and vaccination status."

"Where else could the infection be coming from? Do dogs get MRSA infections like people?" he asked.

MRSA—methicillin-resistant *Staphylococcus aureus*—was an acronym I'd been worrying over since I'd reviewed Grayling's treatment sheet that morning. It was a highly resistant bacterium that didn't respond to conventional antibiotics and could cause overwhelming and sometimes fatal infections in people and animals.

"It's possible," I replied. "We do see it in dogs and cats, although it's usually associated with skin infections or wounds. I don't see either with Grayling."

"Are there additional diagnostics we should be considering?" he asked. "Possibly an MRI or CT scan to identify the site of infection?"

Mrs. Dixon was looking intently at her husband, nodding at each of his questions.

"I know in human medicine advanced imaging is often used in critical patients, but for veterinary patients these tests require general anesthesia, and Grayling isn't stable enough for that right now."

Dr. Dixon nodded. I was relieved that, despite his medical knowledge, he wasn't trying to outdo me, an uncomfortable dynamic I'd encountered before when dealing with animals owned by human—or *real,* as they considered themselves—doctors.

When I applied for university, veterinary medicine was considered the more difficult discipline. Given its James Herriot–induced popularity and the small number of available schools, there were approximately fifteen applicants for every available spot, making acceptance rates much lower than for medicine. And the competition between human and animal doctors continued long after graduation, although the vet student comebacks remain my favorites—in particular a dig so popular it has graced T-shirts: "Real doctors treat more than one species."

Despite our assertion that we were smarter and all-around better than MDs, the human medical profession has, until recently, considered the veterinary profession a poor relative, and even then only by marriage. In my examination room, I'd met physicians who professed surprise that modern veterinary medicine could diagnose and treat their pets, and who, with disdain, elected to pursue what they considered the best course of action based on their experience in the human field.

Although Dr. Dixon's suggestion of advanced diagnostic imaging was not in Grayling's best interest, his comment about MRSA had echoed my concerns that Grayling could be battling an antibiotic-resistant bacterium. She'd received two intravenous doses of a broad-spectrum antibiotic overnight, but she'd failed to respond in any measurable way—indicating that the antibiotic was inappropriate, the organism was resistant, or the infection was so overwhelming that it would take longer for the antibiotic to gain control.

Following the rule book of pure science, I would collect my cultures, await the results of the antibiotic sensitivity profiles, and use this information to guide my treatment. But I couldn't wait the ninety-six hours these results would take to come back. I needed to change the treatment plan—fast—to get a hold on the infection. In the consulting room I tried to keep the urgency out of my voice.

"We'll continue to search for the cause of Grayling's infection," I told the Dixons. "My plan is to perform blood and urine cultures and screen for rarer bacteria. But I also want to focus on her treatment, because she hasn't responded to the antibiotics she's been given."

"Does she still have a fever?" Dr. Dixon asked.

"Yes," I replied. "Her temperature at eight A.M. was 104.3, and she was very depressed when I evaluated her this morning."

"She's quite shy around new people," Mrs. Dixon said. "And with her arthritis she doesn't like these slippery floors. That could be why she's depressed."

I nodded. "Once we've finished here, I'll take you back to visit, and we can see how she responds to you." It was often easier for owners to understand the severity of their pets' conditions when they were faced with the physical manifestation of the disease I was describing.

"We'd like that, wouldn't we, dear?" Dr. Dixon said, reaching for his wife's hand.

"Yes, but I don't want to upset her," Mrs. Dixon said. "I don't want her believing she's going home." Her grip tightened on his, but her eyes were on me. "What do you think?" she asked.

"You should see her." I knew that Grayling could deteriorate rapidly, leaving her owners no time to say another goodbye if she took a turn for the worse. "Would you like to come with me now to visit?" I asked. The Dixons looked at each other and nodded.

I walked slowly from the exam room to the treatment room, the Dixons following behind, their stance erect and somber. Our passage was more like a cortege than a hospital visit. Once in the treatment room, Dr. and Mrs. Dixon bent uncomfortably next to their recumbent dog. They seemed faded, older, in the face of Grayling's illness. I hustled two interns off rolling chairs at the doctors' desk so I could offer the elderly couple a seat, worried for their knees and backs. The hair and splotches of long-dried unidentifiable spills that patterned the seat cushions, which I'd previously paid little attention to, were suddenly embarrassing. I hoped the Dixons didn't notice the mess when they cautiously lowered themselves into the chairs. Once seated, they both leaned forward to touch their dog. I stepped away, trying to offer some privacy, but the regular hospital activity I typically ignored seemed intrusive and loud.

The next twenty-four hours of Grayling's care were outlined on the two-page treatment sheet I'd written up that morning, but the plan would likely change according to her response to therapy. I anticipated that her antibiotic choices and fluid types and rates would need adjustment, and further monitoring, including an ECG and blood pressure, would be necessary if she didn't stabilize by the early afternoon.

The diagnostic plan was also laid out: an echocardiogram—or heart ultrasound—to look for infection of a heart valve; blood and urine cultures for anaerobic and aerobic bacteria; and regular monitoring of her complete blood count, clotting profile, and serum chemistries to assess her body's response to, and gauge the success of, treatment.

I looked over my antibiotic choices again. I'd decided to upgrade one to a potentiated penicillin, increase another to the maximum dose, and add a third to cover for less-common infectious agents. I was pulling out the big guns, something I hesitated to do without a documented reason. I was well aware of the risks of using multiple antibiotics without knowing which was needed; it was this type of practice that created drug-resistant bacterial strains.

Antimicrobial resistance in infectious organisms—including bacteria, viruses, fungi, and parasites—is an emerging and rapidly developing crisis of the twenty-first century. Antibiotic resistance in bacteria has been documented since 1928, only a short time after one of the first antibiotics—penicillin—was discovered. The solution at that time was to develop new agents to outwit the defense strategies of the ever-evolving targets. This proved effective until the late twentieth century and the advent of "superbugs," unwittingly bred to escape the action of antibiotics. The development of new antibiotic classes and new agents within established classes has significantly decreased over the past forty years. Our technology cannot keep up with the genetic machinery of the bacteria we're fighting, and the incidence of multi-drug resistance in previously treatable organisms is increasing.

Blame for the rise of multi-drug–resistant organisms rests uncomfortably on the shoulders of veterinarians and physicians due to their chronic over- and misuse of antibiotics. But they are not the only ones responsible: The use of antimicrobial additives in the food and water given to food-producing animals—to improve productivity and enhance growth at a lower cost—has also been widely condemned. Many of these antimicrobial-containing additives are available over the counter and can be administered without veterinary supervision, a practice that the FDA's Veterinary Feed Directive, released in June 2015, aimed to control. This widespread and indiscriminate use of antimicrobials that are the same as, or similar to, those used in human medicine promotes resistance through prolonged, low-level exposure of bacteria to antibiotics, allowing resistant organisms to flourish once those sensitive to the antibiotic have been killed.

Despite the recent FDA directive, the United States has yet to ban antimicrobials for growth promotion in animal feed, a measure the European Union introduced in January 2006. The U.S. debate about the use, or misuse, of these drugs in agriculture continues to rage, with the economic impact of banning antibiotics for growth promotion trumping concerns over antimicrobial resistance. To put the extent of agricultural antibiotic use into perspective, the Alliance for the Prudent Use of Antibiotics estimates that more than 70 percent of the antibiotics sold in the United States each year are used in food animal production.

The spotlight on antibiotic usage in veterinary medicine falls not only on livestock production. With growing antimicrobial resistance, the treatment of small animals also has come under close scrutiny. Today, the lives we share with our pets are intimate beyond an emotional connection. Beds and couches, counter space for food preparation, and even the plates we eat off are communal among human and four-legged family members. The antibiotics I give my patients, and those used in human medicine, are similar, if not identical.

Methicillin-resistant *Staphylococcus aureus* is one organism that humans and their pets share. Since the 1990s it has been documented in animals at veterinary hospitals, and identical strains have been cultured from human associates. The infection can pass from people to companion animals and, potentially, back again.

Antibiotic-resistant infections are particularly significant in the hospital environment, where pathogenic organisms can gain entry to the body via surgical wounds, compromised skin, or the respiratory, intestinal, or urinary tract. In critically ill patients like Grayling, factors including immunosuppression, multiple antibiotic exposures, and the presence of intravenous and urinary catheters increase the risk of developing a hospital-acquired, or nosocomial, infection.

I knew that aspects of Grayling's care would increase her risk of developing an infection she hadn't arrived with. If she made it through the next twenty-four hours she would likely be in the hospital for several more days, and the longer she spent with us the higher her risk of developing a nosocomial infection.

I maintained a solicitous distance from the Dixons while they visited with Grayling. I could hear the murmur of their voices, but I couldn't make out what they were saying over the familiar noise of the treatment room. They sat doubled over in their seats, with their heads almost touching. Each rested a hand on Grayling and, with the other, clutched their partner's hand. I looked away; even my gaze felt like an intrusion.

"Has she urinated?" Dr. Dixon asked, and I realized that he'd moved from Grayling's side to mine.

I knew the answer—it was a concern I had yet to resolve—but I reviewed her treatment sheet to double-check. "No. Not since she came in yesterday afternoon."

"Is that normal?" he asked.

"I'd prefer if she'd urinated by now," I replied. Grayling was a large, recumbent dog, and her ability to pass urine was a significant consideration. "She was dehydrated, so we first had to correct her fluid deficit, but we should be caught up by now."

"Grayling is quite particular," Dr. Dixon said. "She won't urinate until she finds a spot she really likes. Her brothers will go on command, but not her." It was a familiar observation. Many of my canine patients were fastidious about how, when, and where they would urinate—specific requirements might include being outside, the space and strength to posture adequately, and the right kind of surface.

"Unfortunately, I don't think getting her outside is an option at the moment." I pictured lifting Grayling onto a gurney, wheeling her through the narrow doorways, and then struggling to get her on her feet on the tiny patch of grass, in the hope that she'd like the spot we'd selected. Even if we succeeded, I worried that the stress of the trip could kill her.

"She might be willing to urinate while she's lying down," I said, sounding more hopeful than I felt. We couldn't slide a bedpan underneath her and ask her to pee. The best we could expect was that she would go on the absorbent pad under her back end when she needed to—but I'd had patients refuse urination to the point of potentially permanent damage to the bladder wall muscle. Even if she did ultimately urinate, her fur and skin would become saturated, increasing her risk of developing the canine equivalent of bedsores.

"I don't know about that," said Dr. Dixon. "She's quite fussy about that sort of thing. She's never urinated in the house, not even when she was a puppy." His eyes shifted; maybe he was thinking of Grayling years ago—paws and legs still to grow into, her coat whiskery soft. A tough contrast to the sick, sad dog lying five feet away.

"Given these factors, I think the best option would be to place a urinary catheter," I said. "We can measure her urine output, and alleviate the potential for urine scald on her hind end." I didn't mention the increased risk of developing a hospital-acquired infection with the placement of a catheter. Given Grayling's antibiotic exposure, any bacteria able to survive and set up home in her bladder would be resistant, and virtually impossible to treat. But that was a bridge I'd have to cross if and when we got to it.

I ushered Dr. Dixon back to Grayling and Mrs. Dixon's side. He placed his hand lightly on his wife's back. She sat up and turned to look at us. She tried to smile politely, but her eyes betrayed that she'd been crying.

"Come on, old girl," Dr. Dixon said, bending to help her up. I wasn't sure if he was talking to Grayling or his wife. His voice was gruff, the matter-of-fact veneer fractured for a moment to reveal the worry he must have felt.

The Dixons stood together. "All right, we'll leave you to it, then," Dr. Dixon said. "Not much we can do to help, is there?"

"Can we visit again later?" Mrs. Dixon asked.

"Of course," I said. "We're going to be busy with her most of the day, but we could arrange a visit later on this afternoon or early evening."

"We walk the dogs around five thirty, so after that?" said Dr. Dixon. I sensed the change in his attitude to the more practical matters of daily duties.

"I think that would be fine. I'll have someone call later to confirm."

"Thank you, Doctor. We'll look forward to hearing from you," he said. He took his wife's elbow and guided her out of the treatment room.

The results of Grayling's bloodwork—handed to me half an hour later—revealed a deteriorating situation. Her white cell count had dropped, with an elevation in circulating immature white cells, meaning that her body wasn't keeping up with the demand for infection-fighting cells. Her proteins were falling and her liver enzymes were rising: yet more indication that her body, although trying to overcome the infection, was instead becoming overwhelmed. Most concerning, however, were her prolonged blood-clotting times and decreased platelet count. These changes heralded the onset of DIC. The 50 percent chance I'd silently given her of surviving the infection dropped when I saw the results. There was no time to spare. If I didn't find the right antibiotic in the coming twelve hours, Grayling wasn't going to make it. An educated guess at the best treatment course was all I could make. The time to wait for culture results and sensitivity profiles had expired.

I found Corey at her desk in the corner of the treatment room. I needed to make changes to Grayling's treatment plan before my first appointment, which was rapidly approaching. If I could give Grayling enough time for the new antibiotics to kick in, we might escape the spiraling devastation of DIC that had claimed Fritz.

"How much would a plasma transfusion for Grayling cost?" I asked.

"It depends on how much plasma you're talking about," she said. "She's a big dog, right?"

"Right. She's going to need five units twice a day."

"Ten units, then. Do we even have that much in the hospital?" Corey raised her eyebrows at my gargantuan demand.

"I don't know. I'll check. But theoretically, how much would it cost?"

Corey scrolled through the patient list on the screen and brought up Grayling's estimate.

"The estimate for the next twenty-four hours is almost two thousand dollars," she said. "With plasma it's going to be more like four thousand."

"Okay," I said. "Can you call her owners to get permission for the plasma transfusion? I'll call them later, but I want to get everything set up before my first appointment."

"Sure, I'll let you know what they say."

"Thanks," I said. "I'm going to check our supply."

The in-house lab was situated off the treatment room. There was a fridge-freezer to the left of the lab for storing drugs such as insulin, and plasma in the upper freezer compartment. The hospital's lead technician—Sylvia—was responsible for stocking our blood products, and we usually had a few units available, but depending on our caseload and product availability, our supply could change rapidly. Grayling could use our entire inventory in a day, leaving insufficient plasma for other patients until the next delivery. Sylvia was the gatekeeper of all blood products, and I had to obtain her approval before using any plasma for Grayling's care. I was too anxious to wait for her permission, though, and I sneaked the door of the freezer open to assess our supply.

"I hear you're looking for plasma."

I jumped and turned quickly, feeling instant guilt. "Sylvia, I was just coming to look for you," I said.

"You didn't think I'd be in the freezer, did you?" Sylvia said, a broad grin betraying the sternness she was trying to keep in her dark brown eyes.

"I thought you might be. I didn't see you in the treatment room."

"Did you look? I was fixing your patient's IV. Her fluid pump was alarming."

"Busted," I said. "Okay. I was checking our plasma supply. Grayling needs ten units in the next twenty-four hours."

"You're going to clean me out. Let's take a look at the log."

Sylvia was a lead technician on the emergency service. She also supervised the entire technical staff of the hospital, ordered all the supplies, and performed a plethora of other tasks that kept the hospital running smoothly without most of us realizing what they were. She was about my height with long, dark hair usually tied into a dense, wavy ponytail that attracted the envy of almost everyone. She was admired and respected by the hospital staff, and her integrity was beyond reproach. She regularly got up at four A.M. to bake delicious cakes for staff members' birthdays.

Luckily, the log showed that we had four 240 ml double units and six 120 ml single units of fresh frozen plasma (FFP) in the freezer.

"How long is Grayling going to need plasma?" Sylvia asked.

"Today and tomorrow, if she hangs in. But I'll need more if she's coagulopathic after tomorrow."

"I'll call the blood bank and see what they can send. It's good we have those double units; we don't always get those. If I get in an order by noon today, we should get a shipment by tomorrow afternoon."

"Great. I'm waiting for her owners' approval, but I don't think that'll be a problem."

"Do you want me to check with Corey for confirmation?"

"That'd be awesome. Then you can start her transfusion and order the extra units straightaway. I'll probably be in appointments by then. Thanks, Sylvia."

"You're welcome." Sylvia was already returning the log and heading to Corey's desk.

My last task before starting on my day's consulting schedule was to place Grayling's urinary catheter, which was one thing that was actually made easier by her gigantic size. Finding the urethral opening inside the vaginal vault of a 140-pound dog was infinitely easier than in a six-pound Yorkie. I placed the catheter kneeling behind Grayling, who was lying on the floor, which made me worried that the pants I was wearing would become soaked in urine. I was relieved that by the end of the procedure I didn't need to beg a pair of spare scrubs to get me through the day.

Once my appointment schedule began I would have to rely on snippets of information about Grayling, gathered whenever I entered the treatment room.

A bag of FFP hanging from an IV pole next to Grayling told me that her owners had approved the treatment.

The accelerated coursing of the QRS complex across the ECG monitor informed me that her condition remained critical.

The slow filling of her urinary collection bag with clear, faintly yellow urine showed that she wasn't developing acute kidney failure—yet.

By midafternoon the plasma transfusion was finished, and her temperature had decreased by half a degree. It was too early to say if this was a positive trend or a blip, but the awkward position of Grayling's legs made me think it was a blip. She looked too tired to arrange her limbs more comfortably, and they stuck directly out from her body at an unnatural angle.

I continued with my appointments, torn between my desire to stand vigil over my sickest patient and to take care of those who were less sick but still needed my help. And I hadn't seen Emma all day; by late afternoon I realized she probably needed a walk, badly.

After I finished my last appointment, ensuring that medications had been dispensed and rechecks scheduled, I went to check on Emma, turning left down the hallway toward my office instead of right, toward the treatment room.

"Dr. Fincham?" The voice instantly conjured an image of jet black hair, ruby red lipstick, and a French manicure.

"Dr. Tyler," I said, turning to my boss and feeling, for the second time that day, that I'd been caught doing something I shouldn't. A prickle shivered along my spine; my hackles went up like Emma's did on the rare occasion she met someone she didn't like.

"Heading home?" she asked.

"No. I was about to take Emma for a quick walk. She hasn't been out all day."

"Good for you," she said. Her simper was accentuated by her crimson lipstick. "I'm glad you're thinking of Emma. I've got too much to do to even think of stepping outside right now." I reflected her smile, hoping mine was more convincing. "I've just come from the treatment room," she continued. "Grayling's not looking too good, is she?"

"I've been monitoring her closely all day," I replied, feeling her implied accusation ripple through me. "I'm certainly concerned. She's not responding as well as I would like." I felt defensive.

"Her owner's a retired doctor, isn't he? Not the litigious type, I hope."

"Her owners are very nice and very dedicated to their dog," I said, grabbing my hands behind my back and squeezing, hard.

*Go away,* I thought. *Go away before I say something I'll regret.*

"I'd better be on my way," she said. "More appointments to see, busy as usual. Good luck!"

I turned and continued to the office, determined not to let her see that she'd affected my plan. I closed the door behind me and leaned against it for a second, her "Good luck" ringing in my ears. I took a breath to steady the rage shuddering through me. I still hadn't figured out how to conjure the Teflon skin I needed to interact with my boss and come away unscathed. Emma shimmied across the floor to meet me, her back end, propelled by her tail—which wagged furiously with delight—catching up to her head, so her body formed a U.

I greeted her like always, bending to pet her ears, but at the same moment she raised her nose to lick me in the face, smacking her muzzle under my chin.

"Emma!"

She immediately flung herself, startled, onto the floor, scrubbing her tail vigorously and looking at me out of the tops of her eyes.

"I'm sorry, sweetie. Come here." I patted my leg and crouched down. I felt instant remorse that I'd taken my anger out on her. She got up and slinked half-standing toward me. "Emma, I'm sorry. I didn't mean to shout at you. It's okay." She slurped her tongue across my cheek and continued heartily licking. But I wasn't letting myself off so easily. I rested my arm around the warmth of her body while I considered my options. It was perfectly reasonable to take Emma for a walk. She'd been inside all day, and it'd only take a few minutes. But I hadn't checked on Grayling since before my last appointment. Maybe she'd deteriorated in the last hour. I wrestled for a moment longer, and made my decision. I'd find a technician assistant willing to take Emma out, and then I'd check on Grayling—using the back route to the treatment room so my boss wouldn't know she'd won.

The changes that would indicate Grayling's improvement were subtle. I reviewed her treatment sheet to assess the picture of her day. Her heart rate had remained elevated. Her temperature had fluctuated, but had hovered above 104°F. Her urine output was adequate, but not sufficient to account for all she was receiving, meaning that fluid was sequestering somewhere in her body. I looked at her respiratory rate. It hadn't changed; at least the fluid wasn't building up in her lungs.

I knelt next to Grayling to again perform the ritual of my physical exam. Her gums were florid and her pulse weak and thin, like the pinging of a narrow elastic band. Her limbs had a sickly fullness—the unaccounted-for fluid was accumulating under her skin. She had made little, if any, improvement. A clot of disquiet sat under my diaphragm. Her lack of response shifted the probability of her going home down another few points. Was there something else I should be doing? Something I was missing? *What would Dr. Tyler do?* I wryly asked myself, my earlier interaction with my boss reverberating. She'd shaken my confidence, a familiar consequence.

The Dixons arrived, as scheduled, after their evening walk. I guided them into an exam room to prepare them before taking them to see Grayling.

"How is she?" Mrs. Dixon asked. She sat with her hands gripped tightly in her lap, her feet dangling motionless.

"Grayling hasn't made any significant improvement today," I said. "Despite the plasma transfusion and new antibiotics, I'm sorry to say that she remains critical."

Mrs. Dixon's eyes were too bright in the fluorescent light. Dr. Dixon sat straight-backed, caught in his thoughts of Grayling.

"What else can be done?" Dr. Dixon asked. "We're not ready to lose her." His wife nodded and laid her hand on his. "She's a good dog," he continued. "One of the best. You have our permission to do whatever it takes."

I looked away, but the urgency and desperation of his request trembled in the air between us.

"I understand how much she means to you, and we'll do everything we can," I said. My words felt insubstantial against the weight of their hope. "She'll receive a second plasma transfusion tonight, and we'll continue her other treatments and intense monitoring." I paused. "But despite our best efforts, Grayling may not make it through the night. If she continues to deteriorate I'm worried that she could go into respiratory or cardiac arrest."

I watched their faces, waiting for the impact to lessen before finishing what I needed to say. It was hard to witness. In that moment it didn't matter that the Dixons had spent their lives in the human medical field. Their intellectual capacity to understand sepsis had no relevance. That they had counseled parents dealing with the illness of a child mattered little. They were two people who loved their dog, in the same way that parents love their children, and I was telling them that she could die.

"I'm sorry to ask," I continued. "But, if Grayling were to arrest, we need to know your wishes. Would you want her to be resuscitated?"

"We would want to be with her," said Dr. Dixon without hesitation.

"Of course. We'd do our best to contact you, but sometimes things change so rapidly that there's not time for you to get here. So it's important that we know what you would want ahead of time."

"I see," Dr. Dixon said. He paused, and I saw the effort it took him to keep his voice level. "We would want her resuscitated, wouldn't we, dear?"

The brightness in Mrs. Dixon's eyes turned to tears when she looked at her husband. "I don't know. We don't want Grayling to suffer, do we? Our girl doesn't deserve that. I'd hate to see her tortured."

"We can't give up on her," he replied. "We must give her every chance."

I thought back over the many times I'd had this conversation. In these moments, the unique relationship each owner and their pet shared was distilled down to the most fundamental question of life and death.

"What would you do if she were your dog?" Mrs. Dixon asked.

It was a question I'd once been unwilling to answer, my trepidation at giving the wrong advice overwhelming my knowledge and clinical intuition. But the memory of Fritz, and the suffering I'd witnessed when treatment was pushed beyond the boundary I considered reasonable, impelled me to answer.

"I would let her go. That doesn't mean that's the choice you should make, but if she deteriorates to the point of needing resuscitation I would recommend putting her to sleep. She's been through enough." I felt a beat of trepidation. My opinion was not always welcome, even when it was asked for.

"Thank you, Doctor. We appreciate your honesty," Mrs. Dixon said, a sob, almost like a yawn, stifled in her throat.

"I think we should discuss this further before making a decision," Dr. Dixon said, not looking at his wife. The formality in his voice implied that no further discussion would be had with me.

"Of course," I replied. "Why don't you visit Grayling, and we can discuss any questions after that."

I stepped out to check that Grayling was ready. I sat with her for a moment before escorting her owners to the treatment room, and tried to see her through their eyes. If this was Emma, would I be able to make the decision I'd told the Dixons I'd make? Would I be able to let her go? I liked to think that I would. But could I really know until it was time for me to make that choice?

After Grayling's owners had visited her and had a conversation at her side I couldn't hear, they agreed to a do-not-resuscitate order. Once they'd left the hospital, I spent hours poring over her treatment sheet and rechecking her vital signs. I then rounded her case to the overnight doctors, emphasizing that they were to call me immediately with any questions.

By the time I got home Rob was well established on the couch, looking suspiciously like he'd been napping.

"What's the time?" he asked. "You're home late."

"After nine. I don't know exactly." I peered at the microwave clock. "Ten twenty."

"Rough day?"

"Yeah, I took a sick Irish wolfhound from the emergency room. She weighs a hundred and forty pounds."

"Wow, they're cool-looking."

"I guess," I replied, distracted.

"You want something to eat?"

"I'm good. I don't feel like eating, too stressed and tired."

"Anything I can do?"

"No. She looked so bad when I left. I'm worried she won't make it through the night."

"I'm sorry, hon." Rob patted the couch next to him. "Come here."

Before I could make it across the room, Emma had leapt at Rob's suggestion and was curling herself into a ball at his side, her head coming to rest on his thigh.

"It's okay," I said. "I'm going to bed."

"I'll be up in a bit. Are you sure you don't need anything?"

"I'm good. Love you," I said, and headed upstairs.

Harry, my white and orange cat, jumped off the cat tree at the bottom of the stairs and padded behind me, his presence accompanied by the jingle of his tags. I sat on the edge of the bed to take off my shoes, and he hopped up next to me, extravagantly throwing himself on his side to demand my attention. I smoothed his coat beneath my free hand, drawing comfort from each pass of my palm. It was going to be a long night. Any change in Grayling's condition, or question about a treatment order, would mean an instant phone call, regardless of the hour. I felt a flash of resentment, but I'd moved across the country for the calls, the long hours, the constant caseload. There was no way to escape the hospital. If there wasn't a call I would spend the night awake, worrying about why I wasn't being contacted. If there was, I would spend the night on the phone.

I checked my ringer, turned the volume down to avoid waking Rob, and placed my mobile on the table next to the bed, hoping for a few hours of sleep before it rang.

The closed blind slapped gently at the open window, and the air felt middle-of-the-night cool. It took a moment to realize that I was awake. I instinctively reached for my phone, envisioning Grayling's cardiac arrest, but it was silent. There were no missed calls. Emma was on the floor, gently moaning and sighing her dreams, her body indistinct against the dark carpet. Harry was curled in the warm triangle made by my bent knees, and Rob was asleep next to me. The red glow from the clock on the bedside table set the time at two twenty. There were hours yet until morning.

The threads of my anxiety crept closer—thoughts of Grayling

and sepsis and antibiotics squeezing the remnants of sleep from my body. It was easy to believe in the early morning quiet that I'd missed something, not looked hard enough for the root of her infection, not tried the right combination of antibiotics, skipped a critical step.

Harry jumped off the bed with a soft thud and slinked away. But I was less willing to give up on sleep. Resolutely, I counted backward from ten, but all I saw were Grayling's lab values. Next I pictured myself on a shimmering, deserted beach, but the sand was soon crowded with my patients. Grabbing my phone, I slipped out of bed. Emma lifted her head disinterestedly when I shuffled past, but she stayed put. I headed downstairs to try the couch as a better place to sleep, but I was too unsettled and so spent the rest of the night distractedly watching reruns of *Mork & Mindy*.

I was surprised that my phone hadn't rung that night, although the silence had done little to alleviate my concern. I arrived early at the hospital the next morning, convinced that something terrible had happened and I hadn't been informed. I hurried to resume my post next to Grayling, and while her mortal presence gave some relief, her awkward, still-recumbent position made me question how much longer she could hold on. Her survival for the last twelve hours gave me no hope for the coming twelve.

When I slid my hand between her upper left hind leg and body wall to feel her pulse I noticed that she flinched from my touch. *Odd, that didn't bother her yesterday.* I moved my hand and she again withdrew her leg a centimeter or two. Temporarily forgetting her pulse, I palpated the limb for areas of swelling, or repeatable pain. The region from her stifle (or knee) to her toes was swollen with fluid beneath the skin, which made her tissues spongy and soft. Where I'd examined her leg, my fingers had left small pits, which slowly disappeared when the fluid flowed back to fill the indentations.

I scrutinized the rest of her leg, looking for changes in skin coloration, sensing the firmness of the tissue, the temperature of the surface. And in her calf muscle I noticed a hot hardness. On closer inspection there was a terrible purple reddening of the skin.

"Can you hand me a pair of clippers?" I asked a passing technician.

Tentatively, I removed the hair from the region, careful not to cut her skin. I expanded the tract when I saw the discoloration, like the pulp of a black plum, creeping outward. By the time I'd finished, I'd exposed the skin from above her knee to her hock (ankle)—the intense puce of the central region fading centrifugally to an angry, hot red, and then a ruddy pink.

*So this is what I missed. I should've found it sooner.*

"Make sure you clean those clippers thoroughly before using them again," I said, handing them off to the technician.

The skin in the center of the area looked tight and shiny, like that of an overripe heirloom tomato. I peered cautiously at the source of her infection, unsure what to do next. Should I leave it alone? Stick a needle in it? Send her to surgery for debridement of the area? Amputate her limb?

I decided on a surgical consult, but the surgeon wasn't in until nine. I'd have to wait. In the meantime, I wrote instructions warning Grayling's attendants to wear gloves, and to ensure her leg stayed clean and dry. Then I reconsidered my antibiotic choices.

What were the possible causes of the blooming inflammation in her leg? It could be from a snake or spider bite, although I didn't note any puncture wounds. It could be an abscess caused by a foreign body, like a foxtail, that had become trapped between her toes and then penetrated the skin and tracked up her leg. Or it could be the site of an infection caused by virulent bacteria that had directly entered the skin or been deposited from the bloodstream. None of the options were good. And although I'd found the mystery source of her sepsis I was no closer to finding the cure—if one existed.

In the half hour before the surgeon arrived, I returned to my office to research new antibiotic options. I remembered a recent discussion on the ACVIM mailing list about a potent penicillin-group antibiotic named meropenem, and I decided to focus my search on this drug.

I didn't take the use of such an antibiotic lightly. Meropenem was the biggest of the big guns—a powerhouse reserved for life-threatening human infections—and every time I or my colleagues reached for such an advanced-generation antibiotic, we increased the risk of developing resistant organisms. If meropenem failed to kill the bacteria invading Grayling's leg and bloodstream, I would have not only exhausted my treatment options, but also exposed the microbial population of the hospital to an important antibiotic—a potential problem for future susceptible patients.

I let the idea sit while I considered the rest of Grayling's treatment plan. On review, there was little to be changed from the previous day:

Her ECG, blood pressure, and urine output would be closely monitored.

Her blood gas, glucose, and electrolytes would be checked every six hours.

Her temperature and vital parameters would be taken every four hours.

Her fluid rate would be adjusted every two hours based on her urine output, and her fluid type adjusted based on her electrolytes and plasma proteins.

She would receive another ten units of plasma.

The substantial list of intravenous medications would not change.

Her treatments and monitoring stretched over three pages, but I wasn't sure it would be enough to keep her alive another twenty-four hours.

When the surgeon arrived, we donned sterile gloves and examined Grayling's leg. The surgeon was a middle-aged woman with hennaed brown hair who displayed a brusque attitude outside, and brilliance within, the operating theater. I was hoping she'd provide a smart surgical solution to instantly cure my septic patient. Instead, after prodding the central region of inflamed tissue and commenting, "That looks pretty bad, doesn't it?" she recommended taking samples for culture and cytology—which I'd already planned on doing—and waiting another day or so for the "region to declare it-self." I would add meropenem to my arsenal and wait; there was nothing else to do.

Our hospital didn't stock meropenem because we used it so rarely, so I sent Sylvia to track some down at the UC San Diego Medical Center—the nearest human hospital willing to part with a few vials. An hour later they arrived, and we administered the medication im-mediately, but Grayling was running out of time. She was tiptoeing along the edge of a crevasse, but somehow her feet remained, for now, on solid ground. It would take little—the release of bacterial toxins to cause more inflammation or bacterial emboli showering her kidney or lungs—to tip the balance and for her to die.

Throughout the day I moved between two worlds, shuttling from the relative normalcy of the exam room—and chatting about the best diet for diarrhea or the diagnostic recommendations for a chronic snotty nose—to my critically ill hospitalized patient. I only had to step across a corridor and through a door to be with Grayling, and while I chatted with my clients, a part of my mind stayed with her. Holding the data of her lab results, body temperature, and blood pressure tightly, so I could instantly recall them for comparison when new information arrived, I chased the meropenem into her vein with white-blood-cell-rousing thoughts. I willed her fever to abate, her heart rate to lower. I waited.

Her body temperature two hours after the first dose of merope-nem decreased by half a degree. Was this another blip or was my gust of optimism warranted? I asked my technician to retake Grayling's temperature in an hour. If it was the same or lower, the blip could be considered a trend. If not, I'd have to keep waiting. Despite my inter-nal optimism, I wasn't ready to share my hope with the Dixons. Pre-mature optimism for a critical patient with a capricious disease wasn't a good idea. Assuring an owner of their pet's improvement only to call back a few hours later with news of their deterioration, or even death, was something I knew to avoid. It had almost become a superstition, and I joked that I wouldn't predict an animal's discharge until they were in the car heading home.

An hour later, though, Grayling's temperature had dropped another few points of a degree, and her heart rate had slowed—progress in the right direction. Her left hind leg, however, was deteriorating. A thin, red fluid oozed and slowly dripped from the sites of the needle aspirations I'd taken for culture and cytology. When I bent to examine the skin more closely, I caught the warm odor of rotting meat, but I couldn't discern if it originated from my memory of pathology lab or from my patient's tissues.

I'd called the Dixons earlier in the day to arrange an evening visit. I'd given them a suitably guarded update with news of the apparent abscess and my plan. It was a small victory to have identified the source of Grayling's infection, but that was all I was willing to concede.

By that evening, I felt more confident in the likelihood of Grayling's ultimate discharge from the hospital. I was less confident, though, about her making it home with her leg. With each hour the florid redness had seeped farther under her skin, spreading like fluid blotted with a paper towel. I used a marker to outline the edges of the affected tissue to more objectively measure the infection's spread. The new antibiotic was gaining control of her systemic infection, but poor blood supply to the compromised tissue of her leg could prevent good drug penetration, and allow ongoing damage.

I had to wait and see.

I met the Dixons in the same small examination room as the night before.

"Grayling has made some improvement today. She's not out of the woods yet, but since starting the new antibiotic her temperature has decreased and her heart rate has stabilized."

"Thank goodness. That is a relief," said Mrs. Dixon, the tiny muscles around her eyes relaxing.

"I'm cautiously hopeful that she'll continue to improve, but we won't know if she's in the clear until the next day or so."

Dr. Dixon nodded.

I continued. "Although her systemic infection is improving, I'm concerned about her left hind leg. Has she ever been lame on that leg?"

"Not that we can recall," said Dr. Dixon. "We've been thinking it over since your call this morning, and there isn't anything. No injuries or scratches, nothing."

"I don't know if her leg is the original site of infection, or if bacteria from her circulation were deposited there due to a change in blood flow or a blood clot secondary to her illness." I paused. "Her leg looks quite frightening, so don't be alarmed when you see Grayling. Our surgeon consulted today and recommended keeping the area open, which is why there's no bandage."

"What about surgery?" Dr. Dixon asked.

"I discussed it with the surgeon, and she recommends medical management at this time. Grayling's condition is still very fragile, and we should give the new antibiotics more time. But if the infection continues to spread, limb amputation may be the only option."

The tightness returned to Mrs. Dixon's face, and guilt stung mine—I knew my words had caused her distress. Dr. Dixon cupped his wife's elbow, as if to guide her away from rocky territory. "We put Henry, one of our dogs before Grayling, through that," Dr. Dixon said, shaking his head. "He had osteosarcoma. It was terrible." They shrank closer, withering at the memory.

Large dogs usually didn't do well with limb amputations, especially with advancing age, and six was geriatric for an Irish wolfhound. Saving Grayling and getting her safely into the minivan and home meant also saving her limb—I hoped I could do both.

The following morning, I arrived early to evaluate Grayling. When I approached she tried to lever herself onto her elbows to greet me. Her heart rate on the ECG elevated with the effort. I sat cross-legged next to her head, helping her shift her front legs more comfortably beneath her.

"Hi, Grayling. How are you this morning?" Her head flopped back to the floor, her nose straight between her front legs. "Good girl," I said. "You look like you feel better; how's that leg?"

I continued to speak softly while I performed the physical exam, and I realized that up to this moment, I hadn't seen her as a dog. Her illness had shifted my perspective. Until now I'd seen her only as a sum of organs, systems, and numbers to order and control. I'd wanted to save her because she was loved, because I felt connected to her owners, because they had the money to pay for her treatment, and because that was what I was trained to do. But I couldn't say that I'd wanted to save her for the dog she was—I was only just beginning to understand her as an animal.

While I performed my exam, Grayling occasionally raised her head to inspect me over her shoulder. Her interest was a good sign, and I continued to give her encouragement. I examined her left hind leg last. The skin was uneven with splotches of blackened, irregular tissue sunk slightly below the surface, while other regions looked tense and ruddy. The redness hadn't extended beyond the line I'd drawn the previous evening, but it hadn't receded, either. I gloved up to evaluate the affected area. Her discomfort was clear when I palpated the edges of the region, but the center was less painful; the tissue had already died. I didn't want to send Grayling to surgery, but my unease refused to settle.

The surgeon, however, was unswayed. "She looks better this morning, don't you think?" she said.

"Yes, but that necrotic tissue looks scary."

"Oh yes, there's bound to be tissue death," she said. "But it's better to let her body take care of it. I could make matters worse by going in and poking around."

She examined the tissue, directing her words toward Grayling. "If an area declares itself then I might consider surgery to debride and flush the region. But if we go in, there's not going to be enough healthy tissue to close, and that location won't heal well by second intention."

Grayling wouldn't be going to surgery that day, or likely ever; once the surgeon had made up her mind she rarely changed it. I trusted her judgment, but that didn't stop me from worrying at the decision, prodding at it like she'd done at Grayling's leg, testing it at every opportunity to see if it held.

Grayling continued to stabilize, but she'd been recumbent for three days, and it was going to take another twenty-four hours at least until I was willing to try balancing her upright, on her three good legs. I wanted to be sure her cardiovascular system was stable before it undertook the massive task of getting her giant body moving again.

I tracked her improvement by her response to her owners when they came to visit—the best indicator of how she was feeling in the foreign hospital environment.

That third night she propped herself on wobbly elbows and balanced there for a minute or so when the Dixons entered the treatment room. She nosed her muzzle into Mrs. Dixon's lap once they were seated next to her, and weakly wagged her tail. It was the first time I'd seen Dr. and Mrs. Dixon smile.

The next day I released her from her monitoring devices. The ECG had become a comfort more than a necessity—I no longer needed to see the regular tracing of her heartbeat across the screen to convince myself that she was getting better. It was hard to remove the leads, and for the first hour I rushed to check her pulse several times because she lay so quiet and still. I tried giving her food that fourth day, but she stubbornly refused—turning her head away at the smell of what I offered. It was essential for her recovery that she begin eating and drinking to maintain her hydration and energy levels, but I couldn't tell from her disdain if she was refusing to eat because she was nauseous or because I was the one presenting the food.

When the Dixons arrived with a small plastic container of white rice and boiled chicken that evening, I discovered the answer. I watched from the other side of the treatment room when Dr. Dixon opened the container and held it for Mrs. Dixon to scoop food with her fingers to offer Grayling. Despite their delight at her continued improvement, the weight of her illness was showing through their relief. They hung their heads over Grayling, their gaze intently fixed, willing her to eat. Mrs. Dixon inclined her head closer to Grayling's long, gray snout, and offered her hand with sticky grains of rice on her fingers as if she were feeding a baby bird. Grayling sniffed her owner's hand tentatively. Mrs. Dixon didn't move. Grayling took another second, and licked a few grains from her owner's outstretched hand. I held my breath, willing her to take more food. She nudged her owner's hand with her nose and then lapped the chicken and rice more decisively. Dr. Dixon gripped his wife's hand, resting the container of food precariously on his knee when he reached to pat Grayling's flank.

I turned and left the treatment room before they looked up. This was a moment for the Dixons and the dog they'd come so close to losing.

The next day, the fifth of her hospitalization, it was time for Grayling to stand. Until she began moving, the persistent fluid accumulated in her swollen limbs wouldn't dissipate. And until she could posture to urinate, her catheter would have to remain in place. Getting Grayling to stand on the slick treatment room floor on three and a bit legs seemed as unlikely as a newborn giraffe rising for the first time, and, at the last moment, I decided to gurney her outside to give her a better chance of remaining upright on a surface where she could gain more purchase.

It took four of us to lift her onto a gurney and then wheel her, on a barely-big-enough-trolley, through the waiting room to the front lot of the hospital. Once outside, we lowered her cautiously to the ground and guided folded towels underneath her to use as slings. We eased her into a sitting position with her front legs straight without too much difficulty, and then, with coaxing, brute strength, and a lot of panting, we propped her up on all fours—well, threes anyway, her left hind leg dangling half an inch or so above the ground. We cheered, and Grayling took two tentative steps before sinking again.

I removed her urinary catheter that day. Her only remaining tether was an intravenous catheter, and I was planning on removing that within twenty-four hours if she continued to eat.

The results of the blood cultures I'd submitted at the beginning of her hospitalization came back that afternoon. They revealed that Grayling had a Group A *Streptococcus* in her blood: the type of "flesh-eating bacteria" that caused necrotizing fasciitis in people. I would never know if the bacteria entered her skin, and then her bloodstream, from a small, undetectable wound on her left hind leg, or if she'd acquired the infection some other way. When I searched online and found images of horrific tissue destruction caused by the same bacteria, I realized how lucky we'd been. I couldn't explain how Grayling had survived such an overwhelming infection.

She was ready to be discharged on the evening of day six. She'd continued to eat and drink, and she was getting around on three legs, although her left hind leg still looked like it belonged in a zombie movie. Even though I would be seeing Grayling again more certainly than other patients, like Sweetie, it was hard to say goodbye. The excitement I felt at sending her home was tempered by the knowledge that she may still lose her leg.

After her discharge, Grayling came in daily to be reassessed. Her owners gave her meropenem at home for two weeks, injecting the medication under her skin every twelve hours. Then I switched her to oral antibiotics for another six weeks to eliminate any lingering bacteria. Her leg healed slowly, the skin puckered and tight over the wasted muscle beneath. She walked with a limp, which gradually lessened. New, darker hair grew around the edges of the wound, but in the center, where the tissue was most severely affected, a patch of pale, baby pink skin remained, hairless and soft to the touch.

I continued to see Grayling even months later to ensure everything was returning to normal. The speed of her healing seemed proportional to her huge size—plodding and slow, like an elephant. During one visit, a few months after her hospitalization, I noticed that her heart rate was severely elevated—close to two hundred beats per minute.

She was otherwise well—no fever, breathing normally, good appetite and energy level at home.

*She might just be nervous,* I reasoned, but then why hadn't her heart rate been elevated at previous visits?

I tried to ignore the other possibility—underlying heart disease. After everything she'd been through surely Grayling didn't deserve the dilated cardiomyopathy so common in her breed.

I recommended ECG, chest X-rays, and cardiac ultrasound to alleviate my apprehension.

"Why don't we monitor her heart rate at home first?" Dr. Dixon said. He didn't look at me when he reasoned that she was feeling fine and had no clinical signs—that there was no indication to do any testing because he was sure it was nothing. But Mrs. Dixon remained silent. They'd owned Irish wolfhounds for thirty years, and she clearly knew what they were ignoring. And, as much as my clinical gestalt informed me otherwise, after everything they'd been through I wanted to believe that her high heart rate was merely an anomaly as much as they did. I hesitantly agreed to do nothing.

It carried on that way. Each time she came in I recorded her tachycardia. Each time her owners insisted that at home, on the couch, her heart rate was normal. Surely her heart would've been a problem while she was septic and dying, I told myself. Her echocardiogram hadn't shown any heart muscle thinning or weakness when we searched for the root of her infection. But her heart rate, and her breed, nagged at me.

Four months later I noticed Grayling on the appointment schedule, but not mine. She was scheduled to see the cardiologist. My heart beat faster, and a tangy, bilious guilt instantly rose to my mouth. I knew the precise reason for her visit and I felt inadequate. What I'd dreaded had happened, despite my fervent hopes. She'd seen her regular vet the week before with weakness and difficulty breathing, and she'd been diagnosed with heart failure. Her massive, globoid heart on X-ray suggested dilated cardiomyopathy (DCM), the hereditary heart disease of her breed.

I was angry: This time there would be no saving her. The average life expectancy for a dog with DCM in congestive heart failure was less than six months. She'd survived the odds and beaten a vicious bacterial infection. We'd fought with everything we had. But we couldn't beat her DNA. The cardiologist prescribed medications that might stabilize her condition and improve her quality of life for a few months. But was that good enough? Was that enough for the ten thousand dollars her owners spent? For the pain she must have suffered with the infection destroying her soft tissue? For the days of hospitalization, urinary catheterization, ECG leads, and intravenous catheters?

I didn't know, but a few months seemed insufficient. I wanted more. I wanted years of a good life for Grayling, of trips to Canada in the minivan, of napping on the couch.

But I couldn't determine how long my patients lived. How they would respond to medications. How far their owners would go in pursuit of their pets' health. I could give survival rates and treatment-response percentages, and set the ethical boundaries I would not step beyond. I could improve prognosis with treatment, and I could perform euthanasia when the prognosis became too poor.

But I couldn't predict what would happen next, and whether, after the battle, the journey my clients and their pets had taken was worth it.

# CHAPTER EIGHT

# Ned

The summer of 2009 marked my ninth year in America, and my fourth in San Diego. My visa had become a green card, and my family had stabilized at a husband, three cats, and one dog. My vowels had softened and elongated, and the cadence of my speech had shifted from clearly British to "Let me guess—Australian or South African?" I now called a *moggy* a "domestic short-haired cat" without hesitation. Despite settling in the North Park neighborhood of San Diego, I still considered *home*—the place to which I felt most loyalty and kinship—to be thousands of miles away, across a continent and an ocean.

Even with a family, a mortgage, and all the other small and large things that made a life, I struggled to establish a deeper connection to the San Diego earth. I couldn't find purchase in the sand at Coronado or beneath the ubiquitous palm trees. The sweaters I felt most comfortable wearing lay folded in a drawer; my wellies gathered dust in a closet. But swimsuits and flip-flops were alien to my British spirit. There was no denying my delight at riding my bike everywhere and not needing to pack a raincoat, and outdoor adventures were always a good idea, but I felt a tenuous bond to the place I'd lived in for the longest time since leaving England.

In contrast to my search outside the hospital, the terrain of my veterinary life was familiar. The U.S. units for blood values came to me as naturally as a native dialect, and I automatically weighed all my patients in pounds and ounces. My vet school studies seemed arcane; what I'd once known about horse, pig, and cow diseases was buried under the minutiae of small-animal internal medicine. My world had contracted and deepened like a sunbeam concentrated through a lens. It had been so long since I'd performed basic surgeries—a dog spay or cat castration, or a simple laceration repair—that I felt as qualified to be in the operating room as I did to be on an operatic stage. I could spend hours talking about immunosuppressive drugs, the nuances of different canine and feline endocrine disorders, or the most appropriate diets for inflammatory bowel disease, but when asked about the newest flea preventive I needed to search the Internet.

When I became an internal medicine specialist I gave up puppy and kitten checks and routine visits for vaccinations, ear infections, and itchy skin. And, most of the time, I didn't miss the aspects of veterinary medicine I'd left behind. I definitely didn't miss the glug of fear at the thought of performing surgery. But sometimes, when a dog with intractable diarrhea came back for the fifth time in a month because none of the treatments were working, or I had to inform a grieving widow that her husband's dog—her one connection to her dead partner—was dying of untreatable cancer, I longed for a cute puppy to examine, snuggle, and send on its way.

Unfortunately, a young animal on my schedule usually signaled heartbreak. My juvenile caseload included puppies that weren't growing normally—perhaps due to a congenital, breed-related disease such as a portosystemic shunt, where blood from the intestine bypasses the liver's purification system and instead flows straight into the circulation—and kittens with deadly diseases they'd acquired at birth or shortly thereafter, such as feline infectious peritonitis. My young patients had the types of diseases that carried prognoses expected for animals with their lives behind them rather than in front. In some cases, such as abnormal blood vessels that formed in utero, and conditions like patent ductus arteriosus that occur when normal blood vessels fail to close at birth, a congenital abnormality may be corrected by a several-thousand-dollar surgery, with no lasting health problems. For others, with devastating, incurable diseases, all I could offer was palliative care, which might provide comfort for a few months. The most severely affected, with a poor quality of life and a worse prognosis, were destined for euthanasia. The memories of these young animals, with coats not yet thick enough to protect them from the world, lingered long after they were gone.

Delia, a six-month-old Saint Bernard puppy, was better suited to the pages of a calendar than my examination room. Her coat was soft, with a newly washed vibrancy, the white of her paws and chest not yet stained with years of slobber. Through the fluffy exuberance of her coat I couldn't tell how little she weighed—it was only when I placed my hands on her that I felt her bones pressed beneath her skin.

Her owners were a late-middle-aged couple who had a decades-long history of Saint Bernard ownership. They were both heavyset, with frames that echoed their dogs', and the husband appeared to be growing jowls to rival Delia's. The resemblance would have been amusing under different circumstances. He wore the casual late fifties male uniform of Southern California—khakis, flip-flops, and a Tommy Bahama shirt. His wife was more formally attired, and, when she told me she was a school principal, I wasn't surprised. The tight control she exhibited over her hairstyle confirmed her ability to command hundreds of children. They had recently lost an older male dog and had purchased Delia from their preferred breeder two months earlier.

In the beginning, her quiet temperament had seemed nothing more than a stroke of luck. She was the perfect size for snuggling, and she had an appealing preference for cuddles on the couch over chewing the furniture. Her picky appetite, unusual for a puppy, was also considered a quirk of personality—initially at least. Her owners had diligently weighed her weekly, tracking her progress in a neat, lined notebook, and when the number had plateaued for two weeks they'd taken her to the veterinarian who'd cared for their dogs over the past thirty years.

The abnormal results of her bloodwork had landed her in my consulting room. Their hope was that her elevated renal values were due to a kidney infection. But, after I'd closely studied her lab results and performed my exam, I suspected otherwise. Her thin body, low red blood cell count, and chronic apathy suggested her kidneys were failing for a more devastating and less treatable reason. An infection should have caused a sudden onset of clinical signs, maybe a fever or changes in her urination. But Delia's clinical course had been more insidious, consistent with the slow burn of chronic disease originating from a congenital kidney disorder rather than something more hopeful.

By the time I met Delia, medicine had become woven into my life, and I saw animals, both in and out of the hospital, as expressions of the diseases they might one day suffer. In casual conversation, when the topic drifted to pets, I had to restrain myself from listing the potential genetic pitfalls—of which there were many—of the recently purchased, delightfully cute boxer puppy. I tried smiling instead of grimacing when acquaintances told me of their $1,500 Labradoodle puppy flown in from Florida. I couldn't ignore its potential future orthopedic troubles. And when I saw a dachshund walking down the street, I tried to forget the intervertebral disc disease that was almost certainly in its future.

Dogs have proven themselves to be highly genetically malleable, with a greater than forty-fold difference in size between the smallest and largest breeds, and huge variations in coat color, facial structure, and demeanor, all due to human-controlled breeding. But the appearance of purebred dogs comes with a price. Hidden within the genetic makeup of the more than 350 dog breeds recognized worldwide is the highest number of heritable diseases characterized within a single species.

Strict "breed standards" determined by the American Kennel Club and other organizations specify the acceptable features of each recognized breed, including height at the shoulders, presence of dewclaws, tail length, and carriage, and disqualifying features, which might include incorrect eye color, the wrong shape of nose, or white spots on the coat. These requirements, which run two to three pages for each breed, include more than eighty desirable characteristics that, in reality, are disorders. For example, an open fontanel—or soft spot where the bones of the skull fail to fuse—is an accepted trait in some small breeds like the Chihuahua, and is often accompanied by hydrocephalus and severe neurologic consequences.

The required "adorably" smushed nose of pugs, bulldogs, and other brachycephalic breeds can lead to brachycephalic obstructive airway syndrome—a serious disorder that occurs due to a number of related abnormalities including pinched, stenotic nostrils, and redundant, folded soft tissue clogging the pharynx because the pharyngeal tissues do not shorten in relation to nose length. The consequences include obstreperous snoring, a continual struggle for breath, and a life-threatening tendency to overheat due to inefficient heat exchange in a respiratory tract crammed with awkward layers of soft tissue. In some cases, surgical correction of the abnormal anatomy can provide an improved quality of life; in others premature death is the inevitable outcome. A 2010 report in the *Journal of Small Animal Practice* documented that the life expectancy of the English bulldog was only a little over six years—each one spent struggling to breathe.

Breed-related disorders do not stop at the nose. The spinal column of the miniature dachshund is so long that intervertebral disc disease, with potential paralysis, is close to unavoidable. The English bulldog's head-to-hip ratio is so extreme that puppies can be born only via cesarean section; without human intervention the breed would become extinct.

Beyond the disorders caused by conformation, genetic diseases are highly prevalent in purebred dogs. The University of Sydney's Online Mendelian Inheritance in Animals database reveals how serious a problem human interference in canine genetics has become. In April 2017, the number of known genetic disorders in domestic dogs was 697. The number for cats was 336, and for horses 229. But the most striking indictment of dog breeding is that the number for the gray wolf, their closest wild relative, was six. Human breeding of dogs has evaded natural selection, but not the ramifications of ignoring health in pursuit of perceived beauty.

Hidden in the DNA that gives Cavalier King Charles spaniels their soft coats, liver-and-white coloring, small stature, and charming faces is a deadly heart disease. In 2004, a UK study found that 42 percent of deaths in the breed were due to this condition. Predispositions to blindness, orthopedic disease, and disorders of almost every body system are genetically inherited in many breeds. To date, sixty-three inherited disorders have been documented in the boxer and fifty-eight in the golden retriever. With advances in genetic technology, new heritable diseases are being decoded on an almost daily basis. Until breeders commit to ethical breeding practices and eradicating these preventable diseases, it is likely that my caseload will continue to be littered with the consequences of shoddy genetic manipulation. The price purebred dogs pay for being man's best friend is high.

While Delia waited in the treatment room for her ultrasound, receptionists, technicians, and doctors on other services all came to revel in her cuteness. "What's wrong with her?" they'd ask if they caught me between appointments. I'd tailor my answer based on the inquirer. For those with experience, I'd confess my concerns about her kidneys and the probability of a fatal outcome. But for the receptionists and others less acquainted with the cruelty of disease, I'd chat vaguely, because I knew my consternation would be met with incredulity—they were more familiar with puppies coming into the emergency room for vaccine reactions or with swollen faces from bee stings—and so I chose the easier route. But I didn't have that option with her owners.

The results of Delia's abdominal ultrasound revealed what I had feared—her kidneys were shriveled and shrunken: eighteen-year-old cat kidneys in a six-month-old puppy. Her kidneys had not formed properly in utero, and she had outgrown their limited function by the sixth month of her life. There was little to be done. I could prescribe fluids and medications to improve her appetite, decrease her nausea, and maybe prolong her life for a month or two. I could offer a referral to a university for an experimental renal transplant, which, at the time, had not been performed with any lasting success. Or I could offer euthanasia, knowing that her death was inevitable and that offering a peaceful, planned end might be better than a few months of life poisoned by the toxins her kidneys could no longer excrete.

I called her owners back to the hospital to discuss my findings, a conversation we needed to have in person, though I dreaded it. They'd been taciturn at the initial consultation, and I didn't know how my diagnosis would be met. Later that day, I carefully led them through my findings. They remained impassive. My dread grew. At similar moments with other clients I'd been shouted at, blamed, doubted, or had witnessed the grief of understanding.

"If you decide to put her to sleep," I said, "you could take her to your regular vet, or I could recommend someone who'd come to your home."

"Can you do that here?" Mrs. Church asked. The light reflected off her glasses, making it difficult to see her eyes.

"Yes, we can. You could schedule an appointment with me, or our emergency room is open twenty-four hours," I replied.

"I think we'd like to do it now," she said.

Of the reactions I'd anticipated, this was not one of them. "Of course we can do that," I said. "But you could take her home and spend some time with her before making that decision, if you'd like." Maybe I was trying to avoid the sorrow of euthanizing such a young animal.

"No, we've already discussed this," Mrs. Church said. "We knew something wasn't right, and that she wasn't going to get better. You've just confirmed that for us."

Mr. Church nodded, his expression set. I understood, then, that I'd misinterpreted their sorrow for reticence. They were already grieving.

"Yes, thank you, Doctor, for being honest," Mr. Church said. "We knew something was badly wrong, but our vet kept telling us it was an infection. We wanted to give her a chance, and we've done that. But it's not right to keep her alive. We'd be doing that for us, not for her."

I took a moment to arrange my thoughts. I'd often advocated euthanasia for my patients when their disease was terminal, and I'd seen the devastating consequences of choosing another course, so why was I hesitating? Medically, I knew Delia's prognosis was grave and that euthanasia was reasonable and humane. It was a decision I fundamentally agreed with, but I didn't want to carry it out. *You're being weak,* I scolded myself. *You need to do what's right, not what's easy.* I thought of the times I'd internally railed at people for not making the right decision, and here I was shrinking from my own conviction. Was it because Delia was young and cute that my moral substance was coming unglued?

It was difficult to speak around the claggy lump of guilt—or, could I admit, sadness—that rose in my throat. "I think you're making the right decision," I said. "But I know that doesn't make it any easier." I swallowed hard. I was close to tears, and I'd met this puppy and her owners only this morning.

Their stiffness slackened now that the decision had been made, their tension melting into sorrow. "Can we be with her?" Mrs. Church asked.

"Of course," I replied. "We'll place an intravenous catheter and then you can spend as long as you'd like visiting with her. I'll come back when you're ready."

For the technicians who placed Delia's catheter and drew up the euthanasia solution I knew the decision wouldn't seem logical. It was hard to see why this friendly and adorable puppy was slated to be euthanized. Word quickly spread around the hospital, and I was confronted by the verbalization of the doubts I'd thrown at myself. *She's not that sick, is she? She looks so good. Were her owners making the right decision?* My answers were curt and medical. I'd expended my empathy. *Yes, she was really sick; yes, her owners were making the right decision; and no, there was nothing more to be done.* I took my doubts out on the staff who questioned me.

I didn't know if I was angry with the owners' decision, my inability to save this dog, or my guilt at wanting to do more even though I knew that wouldn't be in Delia's best interest. Or was I angry at her disease or her breeders? Anger and regret were easier to hold than sadness, and I grabbed them when I thought of her lifetime of memories that would forever be unformed. I was used to death, had witnessed it hundreds of times, but euthanizing a puppy never got easier. I envied my surgical colleagues who saved the lives of young animals with fixable congenital abnormalities, and the referring vets who could defer the responsibility of revealing a terminal diagnosis to specialists like me. There was no amount of science or knowledge that could ameliorate the emotion of confronting mortality so directly.

Her owners didn't spend long with Delia before I was called to the room to perform her euthanasia. I was nervous that the sedation drugs might not work predictably given her age, that she might become agitated and excited rather than peaceful. But I needn't have worried. Curled between her owners on a blanket on the floor, Delia died without any more than a deep sigh.

To temper such devastation, and the disorder I encountered at work, my approach to each new patient was routine. I couldn't let go of the seeming order that had first piqued my interest in science and medicine. To combat the chaos, I clung to systematically working through physical examinations and taking thorough histories. I clutched at the semi-quiet of my office, the sequence of my medical records, and the neatness of my paperwork to soothe my turmoil—internal or external—each time I stepped onto the clinic floor.

A typical day began with my firm intention to stay on track and keep on schedule. In the morning, Emma and I would enter the hospital through the back door and sneak to my office, with the goal of going unnoticed. I considered the space mine, but I actually shared it with my boss and the surgeon. They, however, had been working in the hospital for at least a decade longer than I, and had abandoned the office as a repository for moldering memories of medicine past. Instead, they worked from other areas of the clinic. Though their base operations had shifted, they had left behind a hair-coated, fading collection of tchotchkes and cards from clients, yearly conference proceedings dating back to the nineties, and the surgeon's handwritten veterinary school notes from thirty years ago, cluttering every surface I hadn't laid claim to.

One particular morning, about six months after I'd met Delia and her family, I was holed up among the jumble of my office, settled in to my typical task of reviewing the day's schedule. Although I was lucky enough to have a window, the tinted glass and dust-caked blinds absorbed the light from the sunny, blue San Diego sky, making every day look like the end of the world. Despite the hour, the smell of burnt popcorn seeped through the cardboard-thin wall from the break room next door, along with the muted dialogue of a daytime soap opera.

I worked my way through my follow-up appointments, noting the bloodwork or other testing needed for each pet so I could review the day's plans later with my technician, and then I turned my focus to the new patients scheduled for the day.

The first one piqued my interest. He was a young dog named Ned who had a bloody nose. My review of his previous medical record revealed little. Ned had developed intermittent bleeding from the right side of his nose a month prior. He'd undergone treatment with various antibiotics and antihistamines and had had a nasal flush under anesthesia with little improvement. I ordered the notes chronologically, separated out the bloodwork, and considered the possibilities for my new patient.

Unilateral epistaxis (one-sided nasal bleeding) was cause for concern. The list of diseases that commonly caused the problem was short and not particularly attractive, with a malignant nasal tumor and aspergillosis, an aggressive fungal infection, topping the list. I didn't look forward to diagnosing or discussing either, especially in another young dog.

Across the hall from my office was a row of six exam rooms. I could tell, by the particular vibration caused by each door closing, which were occupied. The room closest to my office—room 6—was my preferred venue for consultations, and a familiar resonance suggested that Ned and his owners had arrived. A moment later a technician stuck her head around the door.

"Ned's here," she said. "I'm taking him back for his weight and vitals, if you want to come do your exam."

"I'll be right there," I replied, gathering my white coat, stethoscope, and invisible armor for the day. I preferred to meet my patients before I met their families. Completing my physical exam away from what I imagined was the critical gaze of owners who often wanted to help, or interfere, was easier than trying to perform in front of them. Rectal exams, standing a cat on his hind legs so a recalcitrant right kidney could fall behind the rib cage and be palpable, fully evaluating the oral cavity to ensure there were no tumors hiding under the tongue, and trying to elicit the dance of a complete neurological assessment were all necessary, and easier to do, with the help of a competent technician rather than a nervous, questioning owner.

When I first examined a patient, I formed a picture of their owners in my mind. Grabbing clues from the smell of my patient's fur or the contents of their carrier, I would guess at the type of home they lived in. Sometimes it was easy: the smell of cigarette smoke lingering long after the last puff, or the scent of lavender placed in the carrier to soothe the pet's—or owner's—anxiety. A smudge of pink lipstick on the head of a small, white, fluffy dog accompanied by rich floral perfume was a dead giveaway for an elderly female owner. Sometimes the clues were more temperamental than esthetic. There were the nervous cats whose owners, speaking in a whisper, would hover, wide-eyed and anxious in the corner of the exam room. Or the wild young dogs—often Labradors—whose family, including wild young children, would crowd around the table. Or the skinny, graying but poised geriatric cats, whose dignified owners, suited and similarly elegant, perched on the exam room bench.

These were the pets that mirrored their owners: the pampered pooches with hairdos matching their similarly coiffed humans'— I once cared for an impeccably groomed bichon frise whose fluffed ears poofed from the sides of her head in the same style as her owner's gray-blond hair; the skinny, long-legged dogs with skinny, long-legged owners, both penned in and uncomfortable in the small exam room; and the cats and dogs with obesity, whose owners struggled with the same health problems.

Then there were the owners and pets that occupied opposite ends of the spectrum. There was the huge, confident American bulldog whose energy caused his older, more delicate owner to break her wrist while trying to restrain him; the two-hundred-pound Marine in motorcycle leathers who cradled a four-pound teacup Yorkshire terrier in one huge hand; and Grayling and her tiny owners.

It was entertaining to imagine the families of my patients before I met them, but it was imperative to form a connection to the actual people to understand the animals I cared for.

Experience had taught me to assess a patient's demeanor before approaching them. It was a skill that had saved me from dog bites and cat scratches more than once. After my snap evaluation, I took in my patient's physical condition—watching the rise and fall of their chest before I got out my stethoscope to auscultate the lungs; noticing their position, which might indicate an area of pain; observing their hair coat and fat distribution. I could no longer look at animals any other way. I would analyze the gait of a dog walking down the street in front of me—checking for lameness. Without thinking, I would reach for Emma's pulse while she was lying next to me on the couch, or palpate the saphenous vein in her hind leg to assess for suitability for catheter placement.

Like an excited child who, having learned to read, shouts out the wording on every street sign, I read every animal I met. The thousands and thousands of patients I had cared for taught me how to figure out an animal with my eyes, ears, and hands. It took longer to grasp that I needed to evaluate humans in a similar way. Just as I had discovered how best to approach an aggressive dog or nervous cat, I also had to modify my tone, manner, and vocabulary based on the people sitting across the exam room. I had to interpret their behavior and adapt mine accordingly in order for me to best help their pets.

After nine years of practice, I was less in thrall of internal medicine, and the diseases I diagnosed and treated had become familiar, so I turned my attention to the owners of my patients, and I learned. I learned that, as a doctor, I could choose different ways of saying "I don't know": ways that inspired confidence and respect, and others that garnered skepticism and the loss of a client's trust. I learned ways to ask questions and really listen to the answers, making it clear that I cared about what the owners had to say. I also learned to listen to what wasn't said and to investigate the pauses in conversation to reveal the one piece of information a diagnosis might rest on.

At every exam room door, I took a moment to connect with the version of myself that was empathetic and compassionate, regardless of how those sitting in front of me behaved.


Ned was a small reddish-brown dog, with black tips to the whiskers of his snout. His hair had a wild wiriness that suggested some of his genes were of the terrier variety. His body-to-leg-length ratio was weighted in favor of rooting around under bushes rather than covering any significant distance at speed. I imagined that, if he could talk, his sentences would be finished with an exclamation mark. He was a children's picture book–type dog, whom I expected to get into trouble with strings of sausages, cat chasing, and rumpuses at polite dinner parties.

He was young, about two years old, and his delight at meeting new people made his physical examination challenging; only three paws contacted the ground at any time due to his inexhaustible energy.

On my way to the exam room, with Ned skipping and doodling along next to me, tugging on his leash to get to the next adventure, I pictured his owners—from the pages of the same children's book. A jolly family enjoying long walks, picnics, and romps on the beach.

Entering the room, I was met by two smiling middle-aged women, who both stood up from the bench when Ned yanked his leash out of my hand and bounded across the small space toward them. He thumped his front paws onto the taller woman's shin, and stood expectantly on his hind legs. She bent to pet his head and gently return all four of his feet to the floor before extending her hand.

"Good morning, I'm Karen, and this is Julie. Clearly, you've already met Ned." I shook their hands and met their smiles with my own before inviting them to sit. They were dressed similarly in blue jeans, light hiking shoes, and half-zip fleece sweaters in complementary shades of blue and green. They both wore plain gold bands on their ring fingers, but no other jewelry.

Ned, now off his leash, sniffed around the perimeter of the room intently, scooping up scraps of forgotten fur with his whiskered nose. He sneezed exuberantly and a speckle of blood sprayed onto the pale floor. Julie wiped the splatter with a tissue from a jean pocket. When she looked up I noted the concern in her eyes. "This has been happening more and more," Julie said. "Our floors are covered in old towels to protect the carpet—"

"But we don't worry about the carpet as much as we worry about Ned," Karen interrupted, taking the bloodstained tissue from Julie and putting it in the trash can.

"We're so worried, aren't we, Jules? Our vet said it could be something serious, and we haven't slept since we saw her last week."

"I hope that by the end of your appointment today, we'll have a better idea of what's going on with Ned, and the best way to help him, okay?" I said.

They nodded, Karen's dark curly hair bobbing around her ears enthusiastically. Julie was more hesitant and restrained.

"First, I'd like to go through Ned's history," I said, "get to know you and him a little better, discuss what might be going on, and then talk about where to go from here. I'll start by asking some questions before explaining my thoughts, and then I can answer any questions you have."

Karen began describing the past few months of Ned's life in a tumbling, contradicting narrative. She was clearly excited to have a chance to tell her dog's story. Julie sat quietly by her side, comfortably listening.

When Karen finally paused, I said, "It usually works best if I start by asking some routine questions, and then we can get to the more specific details." I was relieved when they smiled at each other and then me. I hadn't offended them. I doubted it was the first time Karen had been gently asked to be quiet.

My order of history-taking was precise. From listening to hundreds and hundreds of stories, I'd honed my narrative and always repeated the same sequence of questions to ensure I didn't leave anything out.

"How old is Ned?"

"He's about two," Julie said, her voice quieter than Karen's but with a deeper resonant weight that drew my attention. Her hair was the color of weathered cedar, cut to her shoulders and tidily tucked behind her ears. While Karen seemed bouncy and fun, Julie had a seriousness less suited to my imaginary children's book. I'd have to work hard to gain her trust. "Our vet said he was a year old when we got him. But we don't know for sure."

"Where did you get him?"

"We adopted him from Baja Dog Rescue," Karen said. "Poor thing, he was living on the streets in Tijuana before the rescue picked him up. His life must've been awful."

Mexico. I tucked the information into the "important" file in my brain.

"He was so skinny," Karen continued, "but he was such a sweet-heart, we fell in love with him instantly."

"Does he live with any other animals?"

"Our old dog, Maggie, died last year," Julie said. Karen gestured for her to continue. "She was sixteen and she had cancer. We got Ned a few months after we put her to sleep. She'd been with Karen since she was a puppy, and when we moved in together she became our dog." Karen took Julie's hand.

"I'm sorry to hear about Maggie," I said.

"She'd been sick for a while, so it was the right thing to do," Karen said. "But it was still really hard. Now our vet said that Ned could have cancer, too, and we just can't believe it. He's so young—it's not possible, is it?" Both women moved closer together at the mention of cancer, and a hardness, like defiance, crossed their faces.

"I don't think so," I said, wanting to silence the vibrating echo of "cancer," because I understood the terrible significance it held. "But I don't yet know what's wrong with Ned. We'll talk more about that once I can see a complete picture."

I glanced at the clock on the wall above Julie and Karen's heads. I didn't want them to feel rushed. Sometimes I'd joke that my appointments were more like an interrogation, and when I had to flip a question over and over until I asked it in a way my client understood, it did seem a little like a police interview.

"When did you first know something was wrong with Ned?" I asked.

"A while ago," Julie replied. "A month or two before his first visit to the vet. You should have those records."

I looked at the papers on the exam table. "Yes. It looks like you took him in at the end of May, about six weeks ago?"

"That sounds right, doesn't it, Jules?" Karen said. "I think we noticed the problem with his nose in February."

"And what was your concern at that time?"

"We found a spot of blood on his bed. But we didn't know where it came from," Julie said. "When we called the vet they recommended monitoring him at home since he was feeling fine. Then there was nothing abnormal for a week or so."

"We thought maybe he'd caught a toenail," Karen said, "or scratched himself on something. He loves rummaging around in the bushes at the bottom of the yard. But when we looked at his feet we didn't find any blood. We couldn't figure it out."

"Was there anything else out of the ordinary at that time? Was Ned's appetite normal?"

"He was perfectly fine," Julie said, a hint of defensiveness in her voice. "He got up, ate breakfast like always, went on his walk, and chased squirrels. Nothing was wrong."

"Did you notice any sneezing or nasal discharge?"

"No, nothing," Julie continued, the opposition still there. "Of course, he sneezes sometimes when he's sniffing around the garden, but he's so nosy, he's usually just snorted something up his nose."

I knew that it was worry driving her resistance. I understood the need for owners to blame someone, often themselves, for their pet's illness. The questions of what they could've done differently or how they could've prevented their pet's disease were a common part of an initial appointment. My answer was always the same—even if I knew that their smoking had most likely caused their cat's asthma or feeding their dog table scraps had probably contributed to his pancreatitis: *There's nothing you could've done differently; you've taken excellent care of your pet; please don't blame yourself.* Apportioning accountability was not my role, but I'd realized that helping to heal not only my patient but also their owner was.

"How often does he sneeze?" I asked.

"Hardly ever," Julie replied. She had contradicted herself. And I knew that "hardly ever" could mean once a day or once a month. "A while" could be a week or a year. The real answer about Ned's clinical signs likely lay deeper, but Julie wasn't ready to admit it yet.

"Is that once a week? Once a month? More? Less?"

"In the beginning, he was sneezing less than once a month, wouldn't you say, Karen?"

Karen nodded. "But now it's more often," she said. "More like once a day."

"How long has he been sneezing daily?" I continued.

"Do you really think he sneezes that much?" Julie interrupted. "It's not that bad. I've only heard him sneeze once in the past week."

"That's because you're out at work most days," replied Karen, smiling gently at her partner, and Julie smiled back, letting her guard down for a moment.

I was relieved they were smiling. I was often an uncomfortable witness to arguments between partners about what a pet was or wasn't doing, how often it was doing it, and whether or not this con-stituted a problem. I wondered if MDs experienced such disagree-ment in their consulting rooms.

"He's been sneezing daily for the past two to three weeks," said Karen. "He has a short episode after he wakes up or goes outside."

"Have you noticed any blood when he sneezes?"

"Well, that's how we realized the blood in his bed had come from his nose, right, Jules?"

"That's right," Julie said, and Karen jumped in before she could say anything else.

"It was a few weeks after we first noticed the spot. He sneezed and we saw a splatter of blood on the concrete outside, so then we real-ized that the blood must've come from his nose. We thought there might've been other times we weren't aware of, but that was the first time we definitely saw blood coming from his nose."

"It stopped straight away," said Julie. "And after the vet reassured us on the phone, and said it was probably allergies, we weren't overly worried."

I continued to heighten the accuracy of my sketch of Ned's disease, adding color and definition, and the third, emotional, dimension. The good news I would share was that my physical examination had failed to identify the typical changes I associated with serious nasal disease. Ned's nose was a moist, even chestnut brown. Aspergillosis, a nasty fungal infection that, once established in the nose and sinuses, produces toxins that eat through the bone, causes a distinctive depigmentation around the affected nostril—a pale, nude pink against the deeper coloration.

Additionally, the lymph nodes draining Ned's nasal passages were normal in size and texture, and there was no distinctive, rotten odor to his breath suggesting a foreign body lodged in his nose, or an oronasal fistula connecting his oral and nasal cavities, setting up a foul infection. His face was symmetrical, and he didn't exhibit pain when I palpated his facial bones, making a tumor less likely. And, finally, the airflow through both nasal passages was normal, suggesting there was no mass blocking the movement of air. Although I didn't yet know the cause of Ned's problem, I was beginning to drop diseases off my differential diagnosis list. And while the information from his examination and history settled in my mind, one morsel had risen to the top. Ned had been adopted from Mexico, and the diseases south of the border, despite Baja being only a half-hour drive away from San Diego, were different.

Rob and I had ventured to Mexico only once after our arrival in San Diego. Tales of drug cartels, corrupt cops, and the potential for explosive diarrhea after drinking the water had discouraged our traveling there. But when friends suggested a beach camping/surfing weekend on the Baja peninsula, we gave in to our adventurous sides, despite my disinterest in either activity. We drove a short distance south on the I-805 to the Tijuana border crossing.

The San Ysidro border between the United States and Mexico is the busiest land crossing in the world, with an estimated three hundred thousand people passing through the border by foot and motor vehicle daily. Scattered among those entering the United States are dogs, cats, and other animals. Some are pets returning from a family vacation. Others may have been taken to Mexico for more affordable veterinary care. Many are dogs and cats rescued from the streets of Tijuana and the Baja region who are being transported to the States for adoption.

The requirements for importing an animal from Mexico—or any other country—to the United States are surprisingly minimal. Cats do not require documentation to cross the border. Dogs require a valid rabies certificate dated not less than thirty days and not greater than twelve months prior to travel. If screwworm is endemic in the country of origin, which it is not in Mexico, then the animal must be examined and declared screwworm free by a veterinary official five days prior to shipment. Border control has the authority to perform a physical examination to ensure the health of any animal prior to admittance into the United States, but it's not reported how frequently such checks occur.

Dogs imported from Mexico are unlikely to be carriers of rabies: The country is considered free from canine-transmitted human rabies. There are, however, other infectious diseases, typically transmitted by ticks and other arthropods, that can be carried invisibly. These infections may remain dormant until clinical signs appear weeks, months, or even years after the dogs have been adopted in the United States. Differences in climate, environment, and the wild animal populations that serve as hosts for insect vectors all affect the geographic distribution of disease.

In order to diagnose an infectious disease, you first have to recognize the possibility of its presence. Testing for hundreds of different infectious organisms—viral, bacterial, fungal, protozoal, and parasitic—is specific, requiring either identification of the organism or of the body's response to it. There is little, if any, overlap between tests, and selecting the most appropriate, based on history, physical exam, and other results, is essential.

Given the variable geographic distribution of disease, a travel history is necessary to guide diagnostic choices. Without this knowledge, and an understanding of the diseases endemic to the region visited or lived in, a veterinarian may overlook or misdiagnose treatable conditions. This was a mistake I was determined not to make. To lose a patient because I hadn't asked the right question and hadn't looked for the right disease was inexcusable. I'd come close on a couple of occasions, and had only identified the vital information after a repeat journey through a patient's history when things didn't add up and treatments weren't working.

Because Ned had lived in Mexico, the disease that immediately sprang to mind was ehrlichiosis—a tick-borne infection that can cause a decreased platelet count and subsequent nasal bleeding. It was a disease I rarely diagnosed in dogs native to San Diego, but tick infestation, and exposure to the *Ehrlichia* organism, was frequent in stray Mexican dogs. What didn't fit this diagnosis, however, was that Ned's bloodwork had been normal. His platelet count was within the reference range, and his blood globulin levels weren't elevated—often a sign of chronic inflammation or infection. Given these results, it was difficult to justify testing for this disease, and I moved it to the bottom of my differential list.

Ned had finally planted himself across Karen's lap, his nose pointed to the floor like a bored child amusing himself by hanging off the edge of the couch. His back leg rested on Julie—a reassuring point of contact. The women sat with their thighs touching, and they ran their fingers unconsciously through Ned's scruffy coat.

After I'd asked my last question, I saw impatience on Julie's face. I could tell there was something she wanted to say. I noticed Karen's hand edge closer to Julie's on Ned's back. I wasn't sure if the gesture was meant to hold Julie back, or to support the concerns she clearly wanted to express.

"Dr. Jones said that Ned could have cancer in his nose," Julie said. "And we won't put him through a lot. We've talked, and we don't want to spend money on expensive testing if we can't do anything to help him."

I listened to Julie's tone and watched Karen's expression. Had Maggie's illness blunted their tolerance of veterinarians and medicine?

"We know people who've spent thousands of dollars on their pets only for them to die a few months later, right, Jules?"

I forced neutrality into my voice. "Of course, I know how worried you are. But I think that given Ned's age and good health, it's unlikely that he has cancer."

Karen tightened her grip on Julie's hand and nodded, as if in confirmation of what she'd thought all along.

"When a dog has one-sided nasal bleeding," I continued, "it's important to rule cancer out, but there are many other possible causes of Ned's condition."

Karen seemed more relaxed, but Julie remained soberly quiet.

"My recommendation is to perform a rhinoscopy."

"What's that?" Julie asked.

"It's a procedure to look at the inside of Ned's nasal passages. We pass a small scope with a camera on the end up his nose to evaluate the lining and biopsy any areas that are abnormal."

"What do you expect to find?" asked Julie. My answer, *If I knew, then I wouldn't need to look*, remained unsaid.

I shuffled the possibilities in my head. What was I willing to commit to? My clinical gestalt told me I could help Ned. His Mexican heritage nagged at me. What could he have been exposed to before arriving in San Diego?

"It would be uncommon for allergic or inflammatory disease to cause nasal bleeding from only one side," I said. "Most dogs with this type of problem also have nasal discharge and congestion, which Ned doesn't have."

"We looked up nasal bleeding on the Internet when we realized where the blood was coming from," said Karen. "And we kept coming across two diseases, cancer or a fungal infection. What was it called, Jules?"

"It began with a 'P' maybe?" Julie replied, squinting to envision the word.

"Aspergillosis?" I said, relieved that this time "Dr. Google" hadn't led my clients down a completely crazy path. Karen nodded enthusiastically.

"Aspergillosis is a possibility. It does cause nasal bleeding, and I've diagnosed it several times in San Diego. But dogs with this infection are often uncomfortable and have changes in the pigmentation of their nose. I don't see either with Ned."

"That's a relief, isn't it, Jules? That fungus sounds terrible. The pictures of those poor dogs' noses were awful."

"But you haven't told us what it could be," Julie said, instantly sobering her partner's mood.

"There are infectious diseases in Mexico that we don't see in San Diego. Ned may have picked something up before you adopted him, and that's what's causing problems now."

"Really? We've had him for months," said Julie. "Why haven't we seen a problem before?"

"The rescue said he was healthy, didn't they, Jules? A vet in Mexico examined him before he was released, and he got all his shots. Our vet looked him over as soon as we got him, and she didn't notice anything abnormal, either."

"He certainly could've looked healthy and not shown any signs initially," I said. "But sometimes, if the infection is hidden, signs can develop over a longer period of time."

"We thought we were doing the right thing by adopting a dog from Mexico," Karen said. "There are so many strays. And the pictures on the Internet are awful."

I knew the pictures she was talking about. Emaciated dogs shrink-wrapped in their skin, rummaging through garbage to find something—anything—to eat. Dogs curled into cardboard boxes, impossible to tell from a single image if they were alive or dead. Dogs with mite infestations so severe they had pulled, ripped, and scratched out all their fur, their skin rumpled, thickened, and discolored, like the surface of some undiscovered planet. Despite the missing hair, muscle, eyes, and sometimes even limbs, there was still something essentially canine in each picture, the same *dogginess* that has drawn humans and canines together for millennia.

The ethical debate I was unwilling to open with Julie and Karen was one I considered each time I went to Petco. On my way to pick up cat food, litter, or other pet supplies, I'd walk past the playpens of puppies and dogs from Baja Dog Rescue and other organizations that had been set up for adoption events.

The adoption of dogs from developing nations, such as Mexico, Thailand, and India, is becoming an increasingly popular option for those considering a new pet. The Humane Society International (HSI), an animal welfare organization, estimates that the worldwide dog population stands at around 700 million, with 250 to 300 million—over a third—considered "street dogs," without an owner, home, food, or healthcare. It is unsurprising that the average life expectancy of these dogs is less than four years. Improving the welfare of street dogs in countries where the human population endures similar struggles is challenging. Charities such as HSI work to improve conditions for these animals by providing healthcare services and population control in their native countries. Other organizations consider a better option to be exporting dogs and, less commonly, cats, to the United States for adoption.

A valid rabies certificate and a place on a flight—usually funded by the adopter and costing around $300—are the only two requirements for a dog to begin a new life in America, no matter its country of origin.

In 2014, the Winter Olympics in Sochi, Russia, threw an international spotlight on the plight of street dogs. Hundreds of pets were abandoned when their owners were forced out of their homes for construction of the Olympic stadium. Left to roam the streets of Sochi, these dogs were slated for government-sanctioned extermination prior to the opening of the Games. Private contractors killed upwards of three hundred dogs a month until the global media picked up the story, and the force of international opinion demanded an alternate solution. A few Olympic athletes adopted strays and returned with them to their home countries at the end of the Games, and a temporary shelter outside the city, funded by a Russian oligarch and now registered as a nonprofit, housed the thousands of stray dogs that would otherwise have been euthanized. The shelter is still in operation today, and they reported that by the end of 2015, sixty-five dogs had been rehomed outside Russia, costing 49 percent of their budget. Unfortunately, the wider street-dog problem in Russia—it's estimated that thirty-five thousand stray dogs live in Moscow alone—has not garnered the same attention.

Without addressing the factors that drive the massive street-dog population in developing countries, the transportation of homeless animals to the United States for adoption will do little to solve the problem. And the potential trouble for importing countries could be significant. In May 2015, a young female dog rescued from the streets of Cairo, Egypt, was transported with seven other dogs and twenty-seven cats to the United States for adoption. Rabies vaccination documentation was believed valid, and the animals were distributed to a number of foster and adoptive homes on the East Coast.

A week later, the young female dog became sick with clinical signs consistent with rabies. After the dog was euthanized, testing confirmed the presence of canine-variant rabies, and the rescue organization ultimately admitted to falsification of the vaccine certificate that the dog had traveled with. Eighteen people underwent rabies postexposure prophylaxis—treatment to prevent the development of rabies in humans exposed to the virus—once the diagnosis was confirmed. Fortunately, none developed the disease.

Government agencies such as the U.S. Department of Agriculture and the Centers for Disease Control and Prevention continue to tighten regulations for the increasing number of dogs and cats arriving in the United States from rabies-endemic countries, but as the recent case from Egypt demonstrates, the risk clearly remains. Aside from rabies, a reportable disease, there are many unrecorded cases of imported animals carrying other infectious diseases into the country. And the potential for the introduction of diseases previously undocumented in the United States remains a concern.

But we also tend to forget, in light of those poignant videos from other countries, that the homeless pet problem has not yet been solved in America. It is estimated that around 6.5 million pets enter shelters each year. These cats and dogs may be strays, those abandoned and picked up by good samaritans or animal control officers, those relinquished by owners who can no longer care for them, or animals seized as a result of neglect or other welfare violations.

Statistics released by the American Society for the Prevention of Cruelty to Animals indicate that, on average, 1.5 million of these animals are euthanized every year. Some are considered unadoptable due to poor health or behavioral problems, but many are healthy yet are killed due to lack of shelter space and resources. This translates to a vast number of uncared-for, unwanted animals destroyed before they find a home.

Significant efforts are now being made in cities and counties across the United States to end the euthanasia of adoptable animals due to overcrowding and lack of shelter funding.

One solution is to transport unwanted animals from areas of socioeconomic depression, where intake rates are typically high and adoptions are low, to those in more affluent regions where widespread spay-neuter programs and better owner education result in lower shelter entry and higher adoption rates. Even in this model, the transport of infectious diseases along with their cat and dog hosts must be considered.

The displacement of approximately six hundred thousand cats and dogs following Hurricane Katrina in 2005 highlighted the problem of transporting animals of unknown health status, with no veterinary records. Animals who were relocated to rescue organizations across the country carried with them infectious organisms endemic to the Gulf Coast, the most common being *Dirofilaria*, the parasite responsible for potentially fatal heartworm disease. Dogs infected with heartworm who were transported to areas where the disease was uncommon ran the risk of delays in diagnosis and appropriate treatment.

I knew where Ned had come from. I wasn't going to let that information slip through the cracks while I searched for the cause of his nosebleeds.

Surreptitiously checking the clock again, I saw that the hour for the appointment was almost over. To keep my day running smoothly I needed to finish up and have the financial estimate for my diagnostic plan approved. I didn't like keeping my clients waiting, and I knew that an early disruption would result in apologies for the remainder of the day.

"We can schedule the rhinoscopy for later this week," I said, "and hopefully get to the bottom of what's going on."

Karen and Julie turned to each other. "I think that's how we'd like to proceed. What do you think, Jules?" Karen said.

"I think we should see the estimate first. But, yes, that sounds like the right thing to do."

"I'll get the estimate drawn up," I said. "I perform procedures on Thursday mornings. Ned will need to be dropped off around eight, and he'll stay until later in the afternoon, to make sure he recovers well."

"Will he be under general anesthesia?" asked Julie.

"Yes, but Ned is a good candidate for anesthesia. There's always a small risk, but his age and good health make that risk very low. And without performing rhinoscopy we won't know why his nose is bleeding, or what we can do to help. I understand how worried you are, but I think he's going to do well."

Julie looked down at Ned, who'd hopped off their laps to sit expectantly at the consulting room door, suggesting that, for him at least, the appointment was over.

"All right, Ned, we're almost done," Karen said. "Come here, it's not time to go yet."

Ned looked over his shoulder, and then resumed staring at the door, pawing impatiently at the tan paint when it failed to open.

"Ned, you just have to wait a few more minutes and then you can be on your way, okay?" I said and squatted down to encourage his attention. He doodled over to me and began sniffing the pockets of my white coat. "I don't think there's anything in there you'll like." When I bent closer, the head of my stethoscope, which was hanging around my neck, swung forward and bonked him on the nose.

Ned let out a small, surprised yelp and backed away toward his owners.

"I'm sorry, little man," I said. *Great, hitting a dog with a nasal problem on the nose is really going to help the owners' impression of me.*

"It's okay, Ned," Karen said, scooping him from the floor. "It was an accident; you're fine."

"I'm going to get the estimate, and if you have any questions please let me know. Otherwise we'll see Ned on Thursday morning. No food after eight P.M., but he can have free access to water."

"It's going to be a rough morning, Ned," said Karen. "No breakfast. He'll let us know about that, won't he, Jules?"

"He'll forgive you," I said, smiling. "He seems like the forgiving type, right, Ned?"

He looked at me and wagged his tail in response.

"Wait here, and someone will be in with the estimate shortly."

"Thanks, Doc," said Karen. "We'll see you on Thursday."

After I gave Corey the information for the estimate, I headed back to my office thinking about Ned's exploration of my pocket with his nose.

Karen and Julie approved the estimate, and the rhinoscopy was scheduled for Thursday morning. When the day arrived, I was impatient to get started, and hovered anxiously over my technicians while they double-checked the anesthetic protocol and setup for the procedure. Once Ned was anesthetized, I positioned him on his front with his head slightly raised on a folded towel, his nose parallel to the table. I resisted my urge to skip the preliminary steps and immediately scope the right side of his nose to try to determine where the bleeding was coming from. I didn't want to be too hasty and miss something.

I started the way I began every rhinoscopy, by fully evaluating Ned's mouth and pharynx to look for abnormalities that could cause nasal bleeding. I carefully examined his teeth for signs of infection, but they were pristine.

I palpated along his hard palate for areas of softness or swelling that might indicate a mass or site of infection. I looked in the back of his mouth to evaluate his tonsils—small, taffy-pink slivers of tissue peeking out of their crypts at the base of his tongue. Everything looked normal.

Next, I examined his nostrils and the bones of his face again— easier to do when he was asleep and not trying to lick me. There was nothing to find. So far, Ned looked completely healthy.

After I'd completed my examination, I evaluated the nasopharynx— the area above the soft palate that connects the nasal passages to the pharynx. I had to access the region by flexing the tip of my endoscope into a J to hook above the soft palate, which could be a tricky maneuver, especially in smaller dogs like Ned. After a few tries, some muttering, and a couple of swearwords, I positioned the scope correctly. I was looking for masses, polyps, or foreign bodies that could hide out in the small cave, but all I saw was the pink, smooth, normal mucosa, or mucous membranes, of the nasopharynx. There was nothing to indicate the source of his problem. I was starting to feel a little nervous. *What if I didn't find anything?*

Next, I looked directly up his nostrils. Left side first, then right—normal to abnormal—but it was hard not to go straight for the right, where I knew the problem lay. The inside of a dog's nose is packed with intricately scrolled, perfectly arranged turbinate bones. Covering these bones is a thin mucosa designed to humidify inspired air, trap particles and microorganisms, and provide a large surface area for the detection of odiferous particles—a component of a dog's terrific sense of smell. The Italianate convolution of the turbinates is beautiful on a CT scan of a dog's nose, but it's a tight, difficult maze to navigate with a scope only a few millimeters smaller in diameter than a nostril. If the left side of Ned's nose were normal, there would be little to see other than the smooth folds of mucosa crowding the tip of the scope.

After a few minutes of maneuvering around the left nasal passage, trying not to cause too much irritation, I'd failed to identify any abnormalities.

It was time to look in the right side of Ned's nose. I hesitated, afraid that I wouldn't be able to solve the mystery.

I first directed the scope into the lower section of the nasal passage. I inched along, looking for blood or discharge oozing between the turbinate bones—a path to its origin. I'd passed the scope only a centimeter into the nostril when I noted a raised bump of tissue on the floor of the nasal cavity that immediately started bleeding when my scope brushed against it. I'd found what I was looking for, but what was it?

Edging back a few millimeters, I flushed the area with saline to get a better view. When the swirling flames of blood dissipated I could clearly see a small raised mass, like an irregular toadstool head. I inserted a slim biopsy forceps and grabbed a piece of the tissue. An instant swell of blood overwhelmed my view, and I removed my scope to assess the biopsy—a few millimeters in size—before placing it in a formalin container.

The jaws of the biopsy instrument encompassed the tiny chunk of tissue, a small tag poking between the edges of the two cups that had closed to extract the piece. I opened the biopsy jaws and carefully removed the section of whatever was causing Ned's nasal bleeding. I gently rolled the piece across a microscope slide to evaluate the cells—a sneak peek before the pathologist's report came back.

I turned to the technician next to me and handed over the slide. "Can you please stain this so I can decide if we need to get more samples before waking Ned up?"

The technician left for the in-house lab, and I had about five minutes before I could look at the sample.

Blood had begun to slide from Ned's right nostril, pooling on the towel under his head. It was to be expected, but it was still disconcerting. I dabbed ineffectually at the narrow stream and glanced at my watch. While I was worrying over Ned's bloody nose, another patient, Clyde, had popped into my mind, and refused to leave. It was too soon for Ned's slide to have been stained, but suddenly I couldn't wait any longer.

I had examined Clyde a month or two earlier. He was also a young male dog rescued from Mexico, and he had been brought in with blood dripping from his prepuce—the sheath of skin covering the penis. Previous urine testing and abdominal X-rays had failed to reveal a cause. Before ordering an abdominal ultrasound to evaluate his urinary bladder, prostate, and urethra, I performed a full examination of Clyde's prepuce and penis. Circling the base of his penis, at the bulbous glandis, almost out of sight, was a red, ulcerated, cauliflower-like mass. I grabbed a microscope slide and pressed it firmly onto the affected area, hoping to transfer cells that could be sent to the pathologist for cytologic interpretation. With Clyde's history, however,

I knew what I was expecting them to find. I made another slide to look at myself.

After focusing the microscope at 1000x magnification, I peered excitedly at the collection of cells from Clyde's penis. A veterinary cytology book opened to the page on transmissible venereal tumors (TVT) lay on the counter next to me.

Spread across my view through the lens, strewn like a carpet of spring flowers, was a collection of purple-stained cells, each one an almost perfect replica of the one next to it, only variable in size. The individual cells were round to ovoid, looking like perfectly prepared fried eggs, with the deeply hued, indigo nucleus offset from the center. The outer cytoplasm was a paler shade of pinky blue, scattered with clear bubbles—vacuoles. The appearance of the cells was distinctive and definitive. I checked the page next to me to be sure.

"Yes!" I looked up from the sea of cells for a receptive audience. "I knew it. I knew it was going to be a TVT."

I grabbed the closest intern, who also happened to be on the internal medicine service that month. "Come and look at this," I said. "Bet you've never seen one of these before. Come on, this is so cool." I tugged on her sleeve, dragging her with me to the corner lab.

"Look!" I stood behind the intern, gesticulating at the microscope. "Do you know what this is? Have you seen one before? If I told you this came from a dog's penis, could you guess what it might be?"

The intern slid along the counter and turned to me, "Uh, lymphoma?"

"No. What if I told you this dog came from Mexico?" I said. She remained silent. "It's a TVT—a transmissible venereal tumor. It's so cool. Look at those cells—aren't they beautiful? They're just like the picture. I've never seen one before. Have you heard of it?"

The intern glanced behind her, maybe looking for an escape route.

"Um, I think so," she said. "But Dr. Tyler is expecting me in room 5 with lab work. I've got to hurry." She shrugged sympathetically, grabbed a page from the stack of completed lab results on the counter, and scurried away.

Aside from the cells' beauty under the microscope, the canine transmissible venereal tumor is a fascinating disease. It is one of only two known transmittable tumors in the world—the other being found in the Tasmanian devil—and it is the oldest continuously surviving cancer in nature.

As its name suggests, TVT most commonly affects the venereal, or genital, area, and cancer cells are transferred by direct contact between dogs. So, yes, TVT is a canine sexually transmitted disease, curable with a six-treatment course of chemotherapy. It has been almost completely eradicated in the United States due to control of free-roaming dog populations and extensive spay-neuter programs, although the disease remains in remote indigenous communities. In Mexico, the prevalence of TVT is estimated at around 20 percent, and the disease is endemic in at least ninety countries worldwide. The large, ulcerated, proliferative masses caused by the tumor are most commonly located on the genital and perineal area. However, given dogs' social habits, it can also develop in the oral and nasal cavity.

Clyde. Ned. Mexico. Bleeding. Could a TVT grow in the nose?

I hurried across the treatment room to the lab, the memory of the cells from Clyde's sample flashing on my retina every time I blinked. When I got there, Ned's stained slide was still drying, and I waved it around vigorously. As soon as the last water molecule evaporated, I dashed the slide onto the microscope stage. I adjusted the eyepieces, increased the magnification, and looked into the cellular world I'd plucked from Ned's nose.

I took a moment to scan the slide a second time and, satisfied, ran back to the procedure room.

"We've got it!" I said. "We've got a zebra! The sample's awesome. I'm sure Ned has a TVT."

"I'll turn off the gas, then?" my technician asked.

"I'll check his nose to make sure the bleeding's stopped first," I said, moving to the front of the table, bouncing on my toes. "This is so cool! It's something we can fix with chemotherapy—remember Clyde?"

"Ned has the same thing in his nose that Clyde had on his penis?" my technician asked.

I laughed. "Yes. Ned has been putting his nose in places he shouldn't have. I feel a bit embarrassed for him."

I bent to look at his right nostril. The bleeding had almost stopped. "We can wake him up. Just watch out when he recovers. He might start sneezing blood everywhere. Keep out of the line of fire."

"Why?" my technician asked. "Can we catch it?"

"No! No need to worry about that; I didn't want you to mess up your scrubs, that's all."

I was eager to give Ned's owners the good news, but I waited for him to recover before calling them. I also had to remind myself that the owners of my patients didn't always view their pet's diseases with the same enthusiasm I did.

Thirty minutes later, Ned was sitting at the front of his cage barking at whoever passed in an attempt to discharge himself from the hospital.

"What time is he going home?" a technician asked, using the accepted hospital code for *Please get this animal out of here.*

"I'm calling his owners now," I replied, "so within the next hour or two." I didn't wait for a response, knowing that another hour or two of Ned's barking was unlikely to please anyone in the treatment room.

I returned to my office to call Karen and Julie.

"I'm pleased to report that Ned's doing really well," I said after Karen answered and put me on speakerphone so Julie could hear, too. "Anesthesia went well and he recovered without any problems."

"That's a relief," Karen said. "We've been so worried about him."

"Do you know what the problem is?" Julie asked.

"We'll have to wait for the pathologist's report to be sure, but yes, I think we've found what's going on."

"Tell us, Doc. We haven't thought about anything else," Karen said.

"I think Ned has a transmissible venereal tumor in his nose," I said.

There was a moment of silence and then Karen said, "That doesn't sound good. A tumor—that means cancer, right?"

"Actually, this type of tumor is completely curable with treatment, and there should be no lasting effects. It's good news."

"I've never heard of it," Julie said, the formality fading from her voice. "How did he get it?"

"He probably picked it up in Mexico, before you adopted him. It's a tumor that spreads between dogs with direct contact, most commonly during mating. So my guess is that Ned was sniffing a bottom he shouldn't have been."

"Ned has a sexually transmitted disease?" Karen giggled, and it made me smile.

"We need to wait for the biopsy results before we'll know for sure, but yes, most likely he does."

"How do we treat it?" Julie asked. "Can we start today?"

"If Ned has a TVT, then treatment is four to six doses of a chemotherapy drug called vincristine. It's usually well tolerated, but I'd prefer we wait until we have a confirmed diagnosis before we start. We'll get the results from the lab in forty-eight hours, so we can get him in early next week to start treatment. But we'll talk more about that once we have the results."

We arranged a time for Ned's discharge, and a tentative appointment for his first treatment on Monday—if my diagnosis proved correct.

After hanging up I sat and petted Emma. Excitement tingled through me. I would be able to give Ned and his owners a normal life back, free from nosebleeds and illness.

On Monday morning, Ned's biopsy results were waiting on my desk when I arrived. The bottom line confirmed my suspicion—transmissible venereal tumor. I danced happily on the spot. I couldn't wait to get through my morning appointments and share the good news with Ned's owners.

I felt like Ned when I bounded into the exam room, his results under my arm.

"It's good news. Ned does have a transmissible venereal tumor in his nose. We can start treatment today."

Karen and Julie grinned and reached for each other's hands across the exam room bench.

"We knew you were right," Karen said. "Jules and I looked up TVT on the Internet. We don't know how you figured it out. You're like Dr. House."

Ned ran joyous circles around the room in response to the excited tone of Karen's voice.

"I'm not sure I quite live up to his standards," I said, feeling a flush of happy embarrassment. *House* was a favorite in our home; Rob and I never missed an episode. I couldn't wait to tell him about the compliment I'd received.

"You do!" Karen said. "If it wasn't for you we don't know what would've happened to Ned. Our vet had no idea what was going on, and you figured it out straightaway. We're so grateful, Doc. Really, you have no idea how relieved we are."

I beamed. "I'm glad I could help Ned. We've just got to get him through the chemotherapy and he'll be back to his normal self. No more nosebleeds."

"We're going to tell the people who rescued Ned from Mexico what happened," Julie said. "We had no idea there were diseases south of the border that aren't here in San Diego."

"Maybe when we adopt a brother or sister for Ned we'll stick to San Diego dogs. Right, Jules?"

I thought of Emma, my own San Diego rescue, with her broken pelvis and right hind limb that had never resolved. It was impossible to predict the future. Whether we buy them from an expensive breeder with an AKC-registered pedigree, save them from the streets of Tijuana, or spring them from the county shelter, there is no formula—medical or otherwise—to determine the time we have with the animals we love.

# CHAPTER NINE

# Monty

Monty had always been an old cat. I guessed he was eight or nine when I adopted him in Philadelphia. Fred and Harry, on the other hand, were the babies of the family. Once Fred grew out of kittenhood and Harry moved through his lanky teenage phase, the passage of time had no impact on their appearance or demeanor. So it wasn't until I thought about how long I'd lived in America that I realized that my nine-year-old cat was edging closer to nineteen.

I should've been cognizant of Monty's age, but my perception of time had become blurred by my love for him, my first cat. Refusing to confront Monty's advancing years also meant ignoring the consideration of his life expectancy, which was never going to be long enough.

When I asked about an animal's age at every initial examination, I encountered the same irrational condensation of time and memories I was now applying to my own pet. It was a question I asked every owner, despite my evaluation of their pet's dentition, hair coat, and subtler indicators, including gait, muscle wasting, and skin texture, that suggested the age range they likely fell into. The answers were far more revealing than a number. Occasionally the response was succinct, but more commonly I heard a description of how an animal and its people came together.

I'd heard stories of stray cats on doorsteps, in parking lots, and in car yards, and ex–next door neighbors who'd left their pets behind. There were tales of breeders visited, litters viewed, and puppies selected, chosen for the way they'd snuggled into their new owners' laps. I listened to discussions of vacations, birthdays, and family milestones that provided a temporal framework for their pets, whose lives were not measured in the same units.

These narratives were my introduction to the lives of my patients and their families, and I never tired of them, no matter how many times I heard about the kitten that once fit into the owner's palm or the dog adopted at the eleventh hour, ten years earlier, after being returned to the shelter three times by other adopters. Sometimes the story would tumble out in the first ten minutes of the consultation, including information that was more pertinent to an owner's health than their pet's. Other times, the narrative would be more reticent, and it would take several visits before it was fully revealed.

One of my patients was a black cat named Bagheera. He wasn't remarkable because of a deft diagnosis, a lifesaving feat of heroic medicine, or any of the other reasons that had once defined the importance of a case. Rather, he was an old black cat with the type of chronic geriatric disease I commonly encountered. He was longer and taller than Monty, with the smallest patches of white—maybe twenty hairs—dotting his back, but he carried himself with Monty's aging grace. And his owner, an earnest graduate student, didn't seem far from the version of myself who'd taken Monty home.

I saw Bagheera for management of kidney disease and an overactive thyroid gland—hyperthyroidism. I'd treated Monty for hyperthyroidism with radioactive iodine years before in Baltimore when he'd developed the condition.

Over the past thirty years, since its first description in 1979, hyperthyroidism has rapidly become the most common geriatric feline endocrine disorder. It is a modern-day epidemic, estimated to affect more than 10 percent of cats over the age of ten. Despite the abundance of patients with this condition, the cause for the explosion in cases is unknown. Factors including iodine levels in the diet and environmental chemicals and pollutants have been implicated, but their role has yet to be proven. What is certain is that, due to the rising longevity of our pets, the diagnosis of age-related disease will continue to increase.

Bagheera's owner had adopted him from a shelter a year prior to our first meeting, and she'd been told he was nine years old at that time. His clinical signs and physical exam suggested that his age was closer to twelve, but I kept that to myself. While I discussed diagnostic and treatment options for Bagheera, he lounged patiently on his owner's lap. He was a quiet cat, reserving his affections for the person who loved him most. I wondered, as I did for Monty, how he'd ended up without a home. His time in the shelter, likely extended because of his age and coat color, was so long that his previous history had been lost.

"I want to do whatever I can to keep him comfortable," his owner, Leslie, told me. She had metal-framed glasses and long brown hair that was tied back in a ponytail. Her skin was pale, I imagined due to hours spent in windowless laboratories, and her slim build accentuated her youth.

"I don't think he's ready to give up yet, right, buddy?" she said, her confidence growing the more she talked about Bagheera. "And he's given me so much; I want to do everything I can for him."

"It's pretty common to be dealing with more than one medical problem as our pets get older," I said. "Our goal right now should be to get him feeling better, which I think we can do."

"My vet told me that treating his hyperthyroidism could make his kidneys worse. Is that right?"

"Yes, kidney dysfunction is common in older cats, and we often see it in combination with other diseases such as hyperthyroidism.

Sometimes treatment of one condition can exacerbate the other, and lowering his thyroid level can decrease blood flow to the kidneys, making kidney disease worse."

"What can we do? I don't want to do anything that will hurt his kidneys. The last thing I want is to make him feel worse."

"Absolutely. There's a middle ground that may not be ideal for either condition, but is the best option for maintaining a good quality of life. We will need to monitor him closely and adjust his treatments to give him the best life we can."

"So we're not going to make him better?" Leslie's hand paused in her stroking of Bagheera's skinny body.

"We can cure his hyperthyroidism with radioactive iodine treatment. But that will likely affect his kidneys and, unfortunately, short of a kidney transplant we can't cure his kidney disease."

She nodded slowly, her eyes fixed on her cat.

"But the progression can be variable, and some cats can live a normal life. In other cases, no matter what we do, the kidney damage continues to progress. We don't know yet how Bagheera's going to respond to treatment, but we'll get a better sense over the coming months."

I looked at the page of lab results with the most recent assessment of Bagheera's kidney function. My gut told me that Bagheera might have only a year left, but I decided that information was too much to burden my new young client with. Revealing my suspicions would change nothing for Bagheera.

"He's only nine, though," Leslie said. "Doesn't he seem young to have such serious kidney problems? I read somewhere that cats should live to be fifteen or sixteen."

I hesitated. Was I withholding my suspicion about Bagheera's true age to protect my client or myself? No, I reasoned, my honesty would change nothing. Bagheera's kidneys would still be failing; his owner would still be confronted by the death of her pet sooner than was fair.

"You're right," I said. "Cats often live to be fifteen or older, but unfortunately some develop serious diseases at a much younger age."

We continued to discuss the next steps, and with each turn of the conversation I was struck by how much Bagheera reminded me of Monty: The way Bagheera looked at me with an expression close to serious understanding. The snippets of information his owner told me about their life together that so vividly reminded me of my life with Monty. And there also, tugging at the sleeve of my white coat, rising like a palpitation, was the realization I couldn't deny any longer. Monty was old, and I was going to lose him.

I became aware that despite the increasing life expectancy of pets in the States, the number of years an animal had been alive mattered less than the age their owners perceived them to be. And that perceived age, whether older or younger than time dictated, had a profound impact on an owner's diagnostic and treatment decisions, as well as their expectations. In some cases, an owner's belief that their pet was too old for "expensive testing and medication" would result in a terminal decision, despite my assertion that ten for a cat or seven for a dog wasn't old.

The opposite, however, could be equally true and distressing. An owner with a firm belief in the exceptional longevity of their pet, and a refusal to realize that life is ultimately terminal, might demand aggressive diagnostics and treatment regardless of their pet's actual age or prognosis. It was these geriatric animals, with nothing left but the dignity of a good death—hauled through invasive interventions because an owner "didn't believe in euthanasia" or "wasn't ready to let Buddy go"—that caused the most despair. My inability to advocate strongly enough for my patients and wrestle their owners from their denial was devastating. Leading their beloved companions down a futile and painful path was one of the failures I felt the sharpest and deepest.

My proximity to disease and my familiarity with its whims and cruelties did not breach the whisker-thin insulation that still protected me from the harshest medical truths. The good health of those I loved had insulated me from the darkest depths that illness could bring, and I viewed ethical dilemmas surrounding advanced care and euthanasia with the pureness of vision reserved for the most naïve. Although I'd cried over patients' deaths, empathized with owners, and railed against the unfairness of lives taken too soon, the pain I felt had always been one step removed, muffled by the degree of separation that exists between doctor and patient.

By the end of 2009, the only personal losses I'd experienced were the deaths of my maternal and paternal grandfathers when I was a child in the United Kingdom.

My dad's father died first, from a brain tumor. He spent his final days in a hospice I never visited. He'd worn thick glasses with yellowish lenses and had a bald spot that was fascinatingly shiny. Both my grandfathers had served in World War II, as most of their generation had, but it was my paternal grandfather who reminded me most of the soldier he'd once been. He was a BBC *Dad's Army*–type of soldier—sergeant-majorish, but with a comic timing that sweetened the gruffness of his South London accent.

I remember marching in formation with my sister around his living room to his barking: "Left. Left. Left, right, left," stopping only when he called us to "Attennnshun!" Years later, when I rummaged through my grandma's cabinet, I discovered the relics of his life that she'd saved—Chinese checkers that really came from China, the musty khaki hat he'd worn in the Congo during the war—each artifact shrouded in the mystery of a man I'd never really known.

My mother's father smoked cigars and used Brylcreem to slick back his receding metal-gray hair. Even now, these smells transport me back to his living room on a Saturday night. My grandmother would be filling green and amber cut-glass bowls with pickled beetroot, cheese, and sliced tomatoes and cucumbers for supper while we listened to ABBA (his favorite band) and the soundtrack to *The Sound of Music*. The voices of Agnetha, Benny, Frida, and Björn and Julie Andrews always echoed through my grandparents' small council house—which they proudly paid off to call their own.

I remember nights when my sister and I slept over in their spare bedroom and woke to a breakfast of fried eggs, sausage, and bacon, with fried mushrooms and tomatoes on the side. But I don't remember the agony of my grandfather's final days—the colon cancer that left him yellow-tinged and hollow in the bed he'd shared with his wife for so many years. I can easily recall my grandmother's searing sadness, and her anger at being left alone. But the texture of my grandfather's death is vague, smoothed by my mother's reluctance to speak of him and my youthful refusal to acknowledge such serious emotional matters.

When I traveled to the United States in 2000, both my parents and grandmothers were in vibrant health. Separated from my family by thousands of miles, I was distanced from the direct, progressive impact of aging. I missed the eightieth, and then ninetieth, birthday celebrations of my grandmothers. My mum's and dad's retirements. The funerals of distant relatives. Even when Rob's family joined mine, we remained isolated in our San Diego bubble from the effects of familial aging: His mum lived thousands of miles away, in Florida, and his dad had died at fifty, before I'd had the opportunity to meet him. Although death and dying were a constant part of my work life, it was easy to think that they were something that would never touch me personally.

The holy grail of stopping or reversing the aging process has long been a topic of intense scientific research and pseudoscientific theorization. And in the past twenty years, longevity in our canine and feline companions has gained increasing scientific interest. Our pets' shorter life spans allow for more rapid evaluation of the effect of individual factors on the biology of aging, with potential applications expanding to human medicine.

That our pets are enjoying longer, healthier lives is indisputable; a 2015 *Science* article reported that the average life expectancy of the dog has doubled in the past four decades, and that indoor cats now live twice as long, on average, as their feral counterparts.

The factors influencing the longevity of our dogs and cats fall neatly in line with those that influence our own. Vaccinations have decreased deaths from fatal infectious diseases such as distemper and parvovirus; yearly checkups catch problems at an earlier, more treatable, stage; and with highly tailored diet options, disease can be nutritionally managed to enhance quality of life. But the life span of companion animals differs from that of other species in one significant way.

Across nature it is accepted that larger creatures live longer than smaller ones; body mass is positively correlated with the number of years lived. Compare the elephant's decades to the mouse's months. Multiple factors influence this difference, including rates of reproduction, litter size, metabolic rate, and ecologic niche.

Our companion animals, however, break this rule. Cats and small-breed dogs—Chihuahuas, terriers, and multiple others—live significantly longer than larger breeds. As an example, the giant Great Dane and Irish wolfhound typically live a mere six years, while a 2015 International Cat Care study of English cats found that the average feline life span is around fourteen years. And when it comes to small dogs, sixteen-year-old deaf, blind, and crabby Chihuahuas with a grip on life stronger than their grip on my sleeve are not uncommon in my exam room.

The reason for diminished longevity in larger dogs has not been discovered. However, as with much of our pets' lives, human intervention probably plays a significant role, and tailored breeding is likely to blame. Studies have demonstrated that purebred large and giant breed dogs begin aging earlier and at a more rapid rate than smaller breeds—higher growth hormone levels, the negative effect of rapid growth on the skeleton, and the pitfalls of breeding to the extremes of genetic malleability all shape the brevity of the lives of the biggest dogs.

Cats, on the other hand, age more homogenously. Feline body mass and physiology differ little between breeds, and the majority of pet cats are mixed breed or domestic short-haired with an average weight that differs by only a few pounds. For purebred cats, as for purebred dogs, genetic disease can negatively influence life expectancy. For example, polycystic kidney and liver disease in Persians and related breeds, and hypertrophic cardiomyopathy in Maine coons, can result in premature death.


Even with the best preventive care—yearly vet visits, up-to-date vaccination schedules, a nutritionally complete diet, and regular activity—the diseases my patients and their owners faced often disrespected the rules. There was no magic formula to guarantee longevity, just as there was no way to predict how an individual animal and its disease would respond to the treatment recommended in the literature.

When Bagheera and his owner left the clinic after our first meeting, with new diet recommendations, prescriptions to improve his appetite and directions for their recheck, I lingered in my office. My next appointment was waiting, but I needed a moment. Bagheera had given me a glimpse of my own pet through the dispassionate, analytic lens I reserved for the hospital.

I closed my eyes and saw Monty lying in the San Diego sun that patterned our kitchen floor: his coat the same deep rusted brown-black; his body slim, with the paunch of old age resting between his back legs, as if his fat had slid down and collected there. But in the flat light of my office, when I peered at my memory more closely, I realized that he'd become brittle and light, filled with polystyrene. His coat had a tufted, greasy quality that suggested he wasn't taking care of himself, and it was littered with clumps of dead hair—small mats of fuzzy gray undercoat showed beneath the brown-black.

Sitting at my desk I analyzed the increased amount Monty had been drinking over the past months and the way he stumbled sometimes at the top of the stairs after he'd climbed up them, exhausted from the short trip. But then, I reasoned, he was always waiting in the kitchen with the other cats for the tinkle of dry food pouring into their ceramic bowls. He slept through the day, but that's what cats do,

I told myself, given that his housemates, over ten years his junior, were equally likely to spend hours napping on the back of the couch.

I needed to acknowledge that the years I'd once assumed were ahead of Monty and me, which I'd taken for granted, were dwindling to months. His signs of normal aging had slid into indicators of age-related disease.

The differentiation between old age and geriatric-related illness was a common topic of discussion in my exam room. It was a distinction that could be difficult to elucidate and challenging to understand. When did an old cat's napping indicate lethargy? When did a geriatric dog's confusion go beyond cognitive dysfunction and indicate a brain tumor or terminal disease? And if age-related disease was identified, how far should one go to treat it? Was "prolonging the inevitable" justifiable when euthanasia was a legal and humane alternative?

My patients'—and now Monty's—quality of life remained steadily in my thoughts. The oath I'd taken upon graduation—*Above all, my constant endeavor will be to ensure the health and welfare of animals committed to my care*—was a continuing reminder of my duty as a veterinarian. But the purity of that promise was a more complicated and nuanced beast than journals, textbooks, and internal medicine conferences described. It was my patients and their owners who taught me the most about the limits of the oath I'd taken.

When pets become sick and parameters of testing, treatment, and the extent of intervention are considered, the ground becomes boggy. Social, economic, religious, and personal ethical pressures influence the decisions we make for our pets, and the veterinarians treating them are tasked with balancing these factors to ensure their patients' quality of life. But even the quality of an animal's life is subjective and difficult to pin down, especially when veterinarians must make assumptions based on an owner's words.

The human filter we apply to animals—whether they are our pets, those we visit at the zoo, or those who make headlines, such as Cecil the lion or Harambe the Cincinnati Zoo gorilla—influences the way we perceive their behavior and the decisions we make for them. Our desire for our pets to be part of the family, to be our "fur babies," clouds our objectivity in assessing quality of life; what we want for our pets often supersedes the best medical and ethical advice.

The very nature of being an internal medicine specialist, and diagnosing and treating the sickest animals, means I consult with owners who have heightened attachments to their pets. I've met families who don't take vacations, couples who won't spend the night away, people who set alarms to get up in the middle of the night, every night, to care for their beloved companions. Do they make these choices because of the bond they share with their pets, or because of their own needs, or both?

I know owners who have slept on the floor or couch for years rather than leave a pet who cannot get upstairs alone. There have been times I've wanted to say "You don't have to do this anymore; you deserve a better quality of life, too," but I've held my counsel, knowing that the owner was as dependent on providing the care as their animal was on receiving it. The choices we make for the animals in our lives are a deep and entirely personal affair.

We choose our pets. We choose their names, what they eat, even what they wear. We choose if our cats live indoors or outdoors. We choose if our dogs go on hikes or are carried to the mall. And, when it comes to their health, we choose the care they receive and, in many cases, if they live or die.

At Bagheera's next visit he'd gained a little weight, and his owner reported small changes in his behavior that suggested that his quality of life had improved—he was sleeping on her pillow again and greeting her when she got home. But with the news that Bagheera's treatment plan was helping also came a common complaint. Administering the medications was becoming torturous for them both. Leslie dreaded giving the pills as much as Bagheera evaded receiving them.

He hid whenever it was time for his medication, and if she did successfully administer them he would salivate and foam profusely, or spit the pills out after she'd wrangled them through his locked-tight jaws. He'd also figured out that medication might be hidden in his food, and he refused to eat anything his owner had used for drug administration—not a good move for a cat with a diminished appetite.

There wasn't an easy solution. One of the best options was to compound medications into flavored liquids, tiny melting tablets, treat-like chews, or even creams for transdermal absorption. Some owners and their cats have tolerated subcutaneous injections better than pilling. But these options still hold limitations. For most compounded drugs there is little data regarding bioavailability or efficacy, which brings into question whether the desired therapeutic effect can be achieved. And cats might even refuse a flavored liquid or chew, only adding to the frustration. I'd seen owners who would not, or could not, medicate their pet at home, which, ultimately, resulted in potentially treatable diseases becoming fatal.

I'd occasionally had to medicate my own cats, and knew that their tolerance for human intervention varied wildly. Fred, my small, scatty cat, was averse to most types of human contact. The mere act of petting him usually made him recoil. Once I understood his temperament, I'd made him a promise that if he became sick I wouldn't submit him to the same testing and treatment I recommended for my patients. To do so would only satisfy my need to keep him around. Harry, on the other hand, my rock-star cat, was the opposite. He would sit on my lap for hours, willingly submit to nail trims while purring, and allow me to administer oral medications without raising a paw. I'd decided that I'd do whatever it took to save him if the time came.

For Monty, the parameters were blurry. He was beyond the age for the kind of intensive treatment I'd prescribed for Bagheera and other patients. I'd medicated him for minor ailments in the past, and it had been challenging. If he wouldn't take the pill in a small amount of food—which he usually refused after he'd been fooled once—the only other option was to pry his mouth open and shove the tablet down his throat. Unless I hit it just right, which rarely happened, I would leave him cowering and gagging, and me guilty and sorry. Was the benefit of the medication outweighed by the nasty taste it left in both our mouths? My veterinarian answer was yes; my answer as his owner was no.

I talked with Bagheera's owner about compounding medications, and tricks to make pilling easier, and for the time being, she was willing to persevere with the treatment that made him feel better. From the outset, however, there was no cure. The aim was to extend and improve the quality of Bagheera's life, but despite feeding him the right food, administering medications, and, when the time came, giving daily fluids under the skin, his kidney damage was irreversible and progressive. When the best outcome was a life of daily treatment, the objective was less clear. Could I uphold my oath of maintaining my patient's health and welfare while also abiding by an owner's wishes?

The first sign that Bagheera's disease was worsening came sooner than I'd hoped. One Monday morning, only a month or so after his first visit, I took a panicked phone call from Leslie. Her voice was high and tight.

"I'm really worried about Bhaggie," she said. "He seemed a little off last night, but we'd struggled over his meds earlier and I thought he was mad at me. But this morning he's disoriented and confused, and he didn't want his breakfast, even though I gave him tuna, which he usually loves. . . ."

I waited until she'd exhausted her anxiety. I knew that the most likely problem was that Bagheera's failing kidneys had caused severe blood pressure elevation, and he'd lost his sight due to a retinal hemorrhage—bleeding into the back of his eye.

"Can you bring him in immediately?" I asked. I resisted telling her my concern. It was better to wait than to worry her unnecessarily, and I would know when I examined Bagheera.

"I think so. I'm due in the lab at ten, but I can always stay late to finish up the experiment."

"You can drop him off for the day if that's easier," I said, realizing that her cat's illness was only one of many stresses she was under as a geology PhD student. "Then we can take care of Bagheera and you can get to school."

"Thanks, that's what I'll do." Her exhale was uneven. "But I hate leaving him; he's spent enough time in a cage, and I promised him he'd never have to do that again."

I swallowed a gulp of sadness remembering her story of how, when she'd adopted him, the shelter volunteers had tried to dissuade her, saying he was shy and quiet, and not interested in playing or interacting. My guess was that loneliness had driven her to the shelter that day and she'd felt a resonance with the quiet, old black cat. My sadness grew not only from the isolation I imagined she felt and the life Bagheera had led before she saved him, but also from the loss she would inescapably suffer.

"We'll make sure to take extra-special care of him for you," I replied. "You can pick him up whenever you're able."

There was a faint rustle on the other end of the line and a moment's pause, a silence so slight I might've missed it if I hadn't been paying attention.

"Do you think it's time?" Her voice sounded muffled and distant. "I've never had a cat before, and he's been such a great friend. . . . I don't want him to suffer. You'd tell me if you thought he was suffering, right? I'm worried I'm going to miss the signs. How will I know when it's time to say goodbye? What should I be looking for?"

"This sounds like an acute problem. And I'm hopeful we can get him back to where he was. I don't think he's suffering right now, but I'll get a better sense when I see him. I would tell you if I thought he was in pain."

I thought of Monty.

I'd answered the question *How will I know?* hundreds of times, gently suggesting that the decision be made when the bad days outnumbered the good and typical behaviors ceased. The signs of a diminished quality of life were as familiar to me as those of kidney failure, diabetes mellitus, or heart disease.

"But," I continued, "I can't make Bagheera better. And I know his ongoing care is expensive both financially and emotionally. To decide not to go any further is a reasonable choice. I'm here to support whatever decision you make."

"You mean put him to sleep?"

"If his care is becoming too much, then yes, that would be the best decision. Without everything you're doing he probably wouldn't still be here. But there are additional treatments to pursue if that's what you'd like."

"I'm not ready to give up on him yet. I've got to give him a chance. He's given me so much; he deserves that."

I was relieved. I'd soothed my ethical conscience, but the thought of euthanizing Bagheera was too close.

When Bagheera arrived, one glance at his eyes told me I was right. The marbled grayness of his pupils stretched to the margins of his eyelids; only the faintest rims of his irises, slim enough to conceal their true color, remained. High blood pressure had caused bleeding into the back of his eyes, obscuring the light hitting his retinas and causing his pupils to dilate to allow every photon in. If I could lower Bagheera's blood pressure into the normal range and keep it there, he might regain his sight.

Bagheera returned to the clinic daily for the next few days for blood pressure measurement and for evaluation of the back of his eye—his owner rearranging her schedule to bring him in and take him back home before heading to the lab. By the third day of treatment his retina looked more normal and his pupils responded to light. He was regaining his vision. Excitedly, I described our success to Leslie, noting his constricting pupils and normalized blood pressure. I didn't dwell on the medication that had been added to their daily routine or that his hypertension likely indicated worsening kidney disease.

With rapid intervention and careful monitoring, we'd averted the crisis of Bagheera's hypertension, which could have resulted in permanent blindness, seizures, and death. But there was no escaping that his disease was getting worse.

At home, despite occasional glimmers of Monty's old self, the broader landscape of his daily life was growing darker. His hoarse, old voice crying in the night sounded like a lament for an earlier time.

I'd also come to doubt his vision. He could still navigate the house and occasionally landed a well-aimed swat at Emma's nose, but, like Bagheera's, his pupils were shallow, milky pools, and his flame-yellow irises were reduced to a scant rim.

I realized that my cat, who'd survived the streets of West Philadelphia, tolerated a flight across the country while crouched under the seat in front of me, and made it through the addition of a dog to his household, was fading. I'd refused to quantify his decline clinically, so Monty's demise wasn't documented by blood pressure measurements or serum chemistry results like Bagheera's, but rather by the steps he no longer took and the activities he no longer enjoyed.

This was a dichotomy I didn't examine too closely. I could justify the distinction between what I asked my clients to do for their pets and what I chose to do for my own. I was, after all, well qualified to make those decisions. But, regardless of my apparent certainty, when a colleague asked how Monty was doing, I still felt defensive that I wasn't doing more.

Even so, the abstract of *when Monty dies* wasn't difficult to talk, or think, about. The gallows humor that carried me through rough days at the hospital rippled into my thoughts about Monty. *At least we'll get a good night's sleep after he's gone,* I'd say to Rob when Monty's confused, guttural crying woke us in the middle of the night. But my growing concern for my oldest pet was a topic Rob preferred to avoid. Monty was my cat, I was the veterinary internal medicine specialist, and Rob indicated that decisions about our pets' healthcare were best left to me. It was a smart move on his part. He understood that I wanted his agreement, not his opinion, and given that my feelings about Monty swung from grief to denial to optimism, he could never give me the answer I wanted.

When I compared Monty to my similarly ancient patients, there was one outcome I dreaded most—that he would die at home because I hadn't seen the warning signs and had waited too long. His death without my intervention would be a failure. Concurrently, I panicked that I'd become inured to death and would choose to end his life when it was convenient for me rather than at the right time for him. Any decision carried an opportunity to second-guess myself.

Death was the conclusion of many of the relationships I formed with my patients and their owners. Some, like Ned and Sweetie, I could discharge and return to their regular veterinarians' care. But for my geriatric patients, the stepping up of treatments and inexorable stepping down of expectations was a more common progression, with the final act often being euthanasia.

The term *euthanasia* originates from the Greek, *eu* meaning good and *thanatos* meaning death. It is a term that has been part of the veterinary vocabulary for decades, made unremarkable by the frequency of its use—an act made familiar by repetition.

But euthanasia's history in veterinary medicine is murky and difficult to track. Most of the documentation concerns the control of stray and unwanted cat and dog populations over the past one hundred years.

The 2013 American Veterinary Medical Association guidelines indicate that humane euthanasia is best achieved by intravenous injection of an approved drug. And the vast majority of the deaths I've witnessed, and delivered, are a result of intravenous injection of euthanasia solution.

Pentobarbital is the main ingredient. A barbiturate first used in humans in the 1930s to control epilepsy, it is now chiefly used by veterinarians for euthanasia. The solution also contains phenytoin—another anti-epileptic drug—and this combination, at high doses, causes respiratory arrest and cerebral death. Phenytoin contributes to cardiac suppression, and cessation of cardiac activity occurs after brain death. It can be used alone in conscious animals, but today's recommendations, and my preferred method, is to administer a sedative and anesthetic first, to minimize the adverse and potentially distressing effects.

When I arrived in the United States, where dogs are accidentally shot, police carry guns, and capital punishment is a fundamental part of the justice system, I had to quickly establish my relationship with animal death. I was a green intern, and during my first month practicing veterinary medicine I had to euthanize a patient. Without any guidance or supervision, I had graduated from the protective care of Peter and my other mentors.

The examination room I'd used was the largest of the three at VHUP and had a door that connected directly to the treatment room, allowing the easy movement of patients—alive or dead—and making it the preferred location for euthanasia. The floor was gray, the lighting harsh, and the walls cheerless.

I knew the patient, a cat, had been brought in for euthanasia. The owners had signed the paperwork at the front desk, and all that was required was for me to perform the requested procedure.

I entered the exam room, already red-faced, and wiped my palms on my white coat before shaking the hands of the middle-aged couple sitting on chairs pushed against the wall. The carrier, with their cat inside, sat in the center of the metal exam table. I was struck by sadness for this cat who was separated from her owners by a few feet of scuffed linoleum.

"Good afternoon, I'm Dr. Fincham," I said, curtailing my smile into something more somber, which probably looked more like a grimace.

"Good afternoon," the man replied. He was white and heavyset, with a look that suggested he wanted this done so he could move on to something more important in his day, like watching a Phillies game. His wife didn't say anything. She wouldn't meet my eye, and her grip felt weak and ineffective in my hand.

I stepped back toward the table and peered into the carrier to assess my patient. Inside was a petite calico cat. Her paws rested neatly in front of her, and her pink nose and green eyes were just a few inches from the bars of the door. She had a small, beautifully patterned, black, white, and orange face. I hovered, undecided, at the front of her cage. My directive was to euthanize my patient, not to examine her.

"I'm so sorry to hear that Kitty isn't feeling well," I said, trying to catch the female owner's eye.

"Yep, well, the vet said she's got bad kidneys, no cure for that," the male owner said, "and we can't take care of a sick cat, so it's for the best, ain't it?" His arms were crossed over his chest and with each word they seemed to inch higher beneath his chin.

I nodded, feeling certain that Kitty's owners could see my pulse pounding in my cheeks.

"Now, can we get this moving?" he said. "This is gonna be quick, right? That's what they told us."

I nodded again, forcing down the quaver rising in my voice. "Of course. I'll just explain what's going to happen and then I'll take Kitty in the back to place her catheter."

"Get on with it then," he said, turning to look at the wall.

"Would you like to be with her when I put her to sleep?" It was a question I was determined not to forget; to get it wrong would be disastrous.

"I don't, but the wife does, so I guess we'll both stay," he said to the wall.

"Good." I paused, realizing that wasn't the word I'd intended to use in this situation. "So, I'll take Kitty into the back to place an intravenous catheter. When I bring her back, you can spend some time with her, if you'd like, before I administer the euthanasia solution."

"We won't need any time; we've already said our goodbyes, haven't we?" he said, not seeming to expect an answer.

"Okay, then, when I bring her back I'll bring the euthanasia solution with me. You can hold her, or she can sit on the exam table and you can stand next to her."

"What d'you wanna do, Donna?" the man asked, but she didn't speak, only huddled closer to hide behind his broad, saggy biceps. "I guess you can just put her on the table, then," he said. "Anything else?"

"No, I don't think so. Do you have any questions for me?"

"Donna?" Another shrug. "Nah, we just wanna get this over."

I grabbed the carrier and headed for the door to the treatment room, already repeating to myself every word I'd rehearsed and forgotten to say.

In the treatment area, once my hands had stopped shaking and I trusted my voice again, I evaluated my patient for the first time. I wondered, while I pulled her out of her carrier, if I could even call her a patient. And if not, then what was I? Once I had her out of the carrier, I could see that Kitty's coat was sleek, and she didn't have the skinny, hollowed-out appearance I would later learn was a sign of chronic illness. It was my first month out of school, and I lacked the experience and confidence to question her owners' decision. I would do the job I'd been asked to do.

Because the room where Kitty's owners waited was directly off the treatment room, they couldn't have failed to hear her screaming and yowling when we tried placing her intravenous catheter. "Typical calico," the technician said, searching for a cat muzzle and a pair of leather gauntlets to restrain her. "They're all like this, Jekyll and Hyde. Sweet as pie one minute, trying to rip your face off the next."

I nodded, hoping to imply my vast experience with calico cats and my similar frustration, while my hands fidgeted uselessly. I tried to ignore the terrible knowledge that these were the last moments of Kitty's life.

"How much do you want?" the technician asked when she'd placed the catheter.

"Uh?" I replied, trying to remember the recommended dosage of euthanasia solution—one milliliter per ten pounds—and also estimate Kitty's weight.

"We usually use three for a cat," the technician said.

"That sounds right. And what do you normally give as a sedative?"

"I'll get you some thio, okay?"

"Great, thanks," I replied, hoping my relief at getting help didn't sound like excitement.

"Do you want an eighteen-gauge needle or do you want me to dilute it?" It was a question I hadn't considered. "It's super thick, and you're not going to get it through a smaller needle. Some people dilute it; others just use the eighteen-gauge. What do you want?"

I had no idea what to do. A larger-bore needle looked scary, whereas diluting the solution would increase the volume and take longer to give—an idea I didn't relish. "I'll take the eighteen-gauge, thanks." The memory of the male owner's attitude made my decision.

I watched the technician draw up the syrupy solution. It seemed to ooze rather than flow into the syringe. The candy pink of Barbie cars and PowerPuff girls, it was shocking in its joviality. And unmistakable.

Back in the consulting room, I placed Kitty on a folded towel on top of the steel table. I waited for a reference to the tumult I was sure they'd heard, but neither Donna nor her husband said anything. Donna came to stand next to her cat, one hand resting tentatively on Kitty's back, the other grasping the edge of the table. Her husband sat unmoved.

I fumbled the needle of the syringe into the port of her catheter, my fingers slick from nerves. When I grasped her front leg to better situate the needle, she neatly flicked her paw, sending the needle and syringe skidding across the table. The uncapped needle pointed at me accusingly, but I felt only relief that I hadn't stabbed myself or anyone else.

"Maybe she's not ready to go," Donna said, while Kitty wriggled beneath her hand, and I scrambled to grab the syringe and recap the needle.

"We've been through this," the husband replied. "This is for the best, you know it is." I looked down at the syringe wrapped tightly in my hand.

When I asked Donna to hold her cat so I could better secure the needle that would deliver the deadly solution, I was surprised by the tight tang of regret and sorrow that grabbed my larynx. I remembered Peter's words when I was holding a gun to a horse's head: "Don't close your eyes," and I imagined him saying, "For God's sake, don't bloody cry."

I began again, relieved that the interruption would allow me to give the sedative I'd briefly forgotten about. The room was silent, and I wondered if I was the only one holding my breath. I administered the sedative, and the tension in Kitty's body was replaced by absolute stillness. I was barely aware of Donna, whose tears were now pooling on the steel tabletop.

All I wanted was for this moment to be over. I ignored the feeling that I was doing something wrong, that I should've spent longer talking to these people, even though I felt intimidated and uneasy. It was too late, and I was too naïve. And, I realized, if I didn't perform this procedure, I couldn't know what would happen to this small calico cat.

I hadn't yet formulated my script of platitudes to describe the process of death, the soothing words to put a grieving owner at ease and offer comfort. I said nothing. I remembered to listen to Kitty's heart to ensure activity had ceased before confirming her death. I carefully wrapped her in the thin towel, providing some dignity to her loose, empty body, but her head flopped heavily out of my grasp, and she began to leak urine, which trickled warmly down the front of my white coat. I exited the exam room with an inelegant urgency and laid her on an empty table in the treatment room. I held my tears until I escaped to the nearest bathroom.

The position pets occupy in our lives strongly influences our decisions, as owners, about end-of-life care. Although, legally, our pets are property, it is now common to view our animal and human families as one and the same, and the role pets play is rapidly evolving. Health-care by proxy—making decisions for those who cannot speak or decide for themselves—is increasingly a facet of modern human medicine, although it has always been a part of veterinary medicine. The questions surrounding how much to do and how far to go for our pets are equally relevant to the choices we must make for our human loved ones. With an aging population and advances in health-care that can prolong life further than at any other time in history, we confront the same decisions for our parents, grandparents, spouses, and partners who are no longer able to influence the course of their care at the end of their lives.

The often-wished-for fairy-tale ending of passing away peacefully during sleep, is, in my experience, a rare reality. The death I've witnessed has not been so considerate. The terminal consequences of the diseases I treat include uncontrolled bleeding, seizures from end-stage liver or kidney disease, and suffocation due to fluid accumulation in or around the lungs, none of which result in a quiet, clean, passive death. Euthanasia, on the other hand, with the careful administration of sequential drugs through a securely placed intravenous catheter, can provide the pain-free, dignified end so many of us seek, not only for our pets but also for ourselves. The pain from euthanasia stems not from the process itself, but from the decision to pursue the course.

While Bagheera continued to maintain his kidney function without exhibiting the dire symptoms that hypertension predicted, Monty continued his inexorable decline. We approached and hovered just above the line I'd set for Monty's quality of life—when he no longer wanted to eat, when he couldn't use the litter box—and he continued to move parallel to it, never crossing over. *How long can we live like this?* I wondered.

These were questions I was able to avoid with Bagheera's owner.

His blood pressure remained stable, he'd called a truce over receiving medications, and his appetite was good. For now, we could expect to measure his life in months to years, but my old black cat was down to weeks or days.

The morning Monty was too weak to get off his bed was no easier because of its inevitability. I brought him a bowl of Fancy Feast, the go-to kitty comfort food that could usually entice the most reluctant eater. It had been his staple diet for the past few months, but that morning he wasn't interested. I lifted him up, acutely aware of his fragility—the hollowness of a body barely occupied.

Rob drove us to the hospital. I cradled Monty on my lap, running my hand over and over his body. Memories swirled around me:

Carrying Monty home down Baltimore Avenue, the sound of his meow filling my ears.

The half-eaten mouse I'd found in the closet in my tiny room in Philadelphia.

The tears his coat had absorbed and the loneliness he'd eased when a solitary weekend in an unfamiliar city stretched before me.

The road trips we'd taken with him screaming his discontent from the backseat.

I felt the weight of his body on my shoulders when he would wrap himself around the back of my neck like a scarf. He was so light now on my lap.

It was easier to think of everything that had been rather than to contemplate what was to come.

For the first time I stepped into the hospital as a client and checked in at the front desk, registering Monty as a patient. I skipped the waiting room and took him directly to the treatment room, Rob walking a pace behind. The ER vet on duty knew we were on our way, and the catheter setup had been arranged. I noted the familiar fringe of tape attached to the edge of the treatment table when I calmly handed Monty to Sylvia. It was a small comfort that she would be the one placing his catheter. She would be careful when probing his fragile veins.

Rob and I sat in an exam room. I couldn't stem the flood of thoughts of Monty. The smell of his breath, the leathery softness of his paw pads, his peculiar likes and dislikes. He'd been the one constant in my life since my arrival in America—and soon he would be gone. There was a surreal distance that separated my love for him—which should've protected him from anything—and the blue vinyl bench we sat on. I couldn't see beyond my memories, and I didn't want to.

Sylvia brought Monty into the room. He was wrapped in a fleecy blue blanket, and his catheterized leg was hidden beneath the fabric.

"Would you like some time with him?" Sylvia asked. A question I'd asked more times than I could count.

I looked to Rob for an answer. I felt paralyzed and unqualified. "It's up to you, honey, whatever you prefer," he replied to my silent question.

"Just a few minutes," I said, the knot of grief I'd been holding tightly unraveling with the words.

Sylvia nodded and handed Monty to me with the reverence of a religious relic, but he felt awkward and foreign in my arms. I'd lost an essential part of him, of the reference point between us, when I registered him as a patient. I was not a doctor, and I didn't know what to do.

I trembled with the effort of keeping my emotions contained. I was shy and embarrassed in front of Rob and in this exam room that had remained separate from my personal life, until now. Rob was the person who knew me most deeply, but there was something different I'd shared with Monty that I was about to lose.

When the ER vet entered the room, the minutes I'd spent with Monty felt insubstantial even though they'd seemed unending when they were passing. I wanted to change my mind, pretend there was a misunderstanding, but I knew I would do neither.

"Are you ready?" the vet asked. I nodded, tears now dripping from my chin and rolling down Monty's faded coat like they'd done so many times before. I told him I loved him and kissed the back of his head, burying my face for a moment in his neck. I shifted him more comfortably on my lap. I couldn't breathe.

I knew the technicalities of what was coming. First, flush the catheter with saline, then administer an anesthetic, and finally, when Monty was asleep, deliver the euthanasia solution. He would likely stop breathing once the anesthetic had been given, and his heartbeat would fade to silence while the euthanasia solution was administered. I'd heard the moment of death; the faraway sound of each pulse getting fainter and fainter until a muffled silence, and maybe the crackle of fur against the stethoscope diaphragm, was all that filtered into my ears. Like a train passing down a tunnel into the distance.

I continued petting him and telling him that I loved him. Willing his passing to be peaceful, racked with a guilt that now, at the end, the life we'd shared had not been good enough. I panicked at the thought that what I'd given him was insufficient compared to what he'd given me. That in this final moment I'd failed in the reckoning.

When the vet stood up from kneeling on the floor before me, Monty was gone. I didn't need her to listen to his chest to tell me so. His weight was flaccid. He felt like he would melt through the blanket and onto the floor. There was nothing holding him together.

"Would you like a few minutes?" she asked.

"Just a few," I said, unable to look up.

I gripped Monty tightly in the blanket, scared I would drop his body.

I'd made the right decision.

I hadn't let Monty suffer because I couldn't bear to let him go.

But this did nothing to ease my sorrow.

I'd never experienced this deep a loss before. And I saw, for the first time, the full expanse of the gulf I'd stepped across when I transformed from veterinarian to owner.

# Epilogue

## JULY 2016

I've dedicated the last twenty-six years to the anatomy, physiology, pathophysiology, and medicine of dogs and cats. I can tell you the receptor a steroid binds to and what it does in the body, why lilies are poisonous to cats and chocolate toxic to dogs. I know which cells do what in the kidney, liver, and intestine. If I close my eyes I can see them through the eyepiece of a microscope—the villi protruding from the intestinal border, a coral reef caught in paraffin; the tessellating perfection of blue hepatocytes; the stout, soldier-like uniformity of the kidneys' glomerular membrane, the cells standing shoulder to shoulder.

I've diagnosed cancer of almost every organ; bacterial, fungal, and viral infections; diabetes, kidney failure, liver failure, heart failure. I've prescribed antibiotics, chemotherapy agents, pain medication, and hundreds of other drugs. I have listened to stories, so many stories. Stories of life and stories of what is soon to be death; stories of tiny kittens grown into old, frail cats; rambunctious puppies grown into arthritic geriatrics.

I hear myself saying, "Dogs are so bad at telling us when they are sick. Often, by the time we know something is wrong, there's nothing we can do."

I have held people's hearts, hopes, and fears when I gently described a diagnosis, prognosis, and options.

I've held hands while delivering the news *There is nothing more we can do,* and the advice *When the bad times outweigh the good, then it's time.*

I have held my breath and held back tears while administering euthanasia solution to a beloved companion, knowing in that instant that the moment has become a waypoint in the life of that family. I've experienced time and time again the deep, inexplicable bond we have with our pets.

I have always—almost always—had an answer for the seemingly unanswerable. A solution to the riddle, a diagnosis to piece the puzzle of clinical signs together. *We were at the park yesterday. She ate her breakfast. He seemed fine,* and then: *What could I have done differently? What am I going to do now? The house will seem so empty. How can this piece of my heart, hidden inside the coat, skin, and bones of a cat, be gone?*

I've been heroic, optimistic, pessimistic, and realistic. I've cried for my patients and their families while my own pain was softened by the sterile words of a diagnosis.

I have been a veterinarian in every waking and sleeping moment— in the hospital, in my car, in my home—my brain rattling through lists of patients and their problems, my anxieties infiltrating my family. Yet, when I lost Monty, and then a year later, Fred, and then, two years after that, Harry, my veterinary experience did nothing to dissolve the crystalline hardness of my grief.

On a typically glorious San Diego day two years ago, I took Emma to our local dog wash. We walked, Emma dawdling to smell every inch of pavement and greet everyone we passed, way more interested in the humans than their canine companions. Emma preferred life at a slow pace. The back right leg she'd had surgery on years earlier— the reason for our first meeting—had never fully recovered, and she still had that slight limp. The scar on her right thigh was still visible when the light hit her fur at the right angle.

Over the previous year, her face had grayed, and she now had the white muzzle and eyebrows of age and wisdom. Even the tips of her toes were white, a snowy fringe around each paw pad. She didn't particularly enjoy baths, but given that her favorite place to sleep was snuggled on the couch between Rob and me, an occasional scrub to remove the carpet of hair she shed around the house and freshen her up was required.

On arrival at the dog wash I lifted Emma into the tub, swearing that she'd gained ten pounds since the last time I'd picked her up. Once she was safely deposited into the deep basin, she hung her head and fixed me with a look of disgusted displeasure that could only be described as "hangdog." I turned on the water, adjusted the temperature, and began spraying her body, watching the droplets shimmer and roll off her oily coat like she was a seabird.

I ran my hand over her back and legs, encouraging the water to penetrate her thick outer coat. I gently directed the stream over her head and neck and worked backward toward her front legs and shoulders. Music was playing through the shop speakers, an eighties channel, and the air was filled with the pungent humidity of wet dogs and shampoo. It was satisfying and soothing to see the water blacken her fur, to feel handfuls of hair shed from her body. When a-ha's "Take On Me" came on the radio, I smiled, reminded of when my sister had bought the album on cassette tape and listened to it over and over.

I sang along in my head, absently washing Emma's neck and shoulders, and while I thought of the music we listened to in the backseat of our red Vauxhall Astra on family holidays, my palm passed over a hard irregularity in front of Emma's left shoulder. A perfect drop of fear slid into my stomach. The music stopped. I ran my hand over the region again, slower this time, more cautiously. The fear curdled and grew, like egg white in boiling water. There was a mass. A firm, fixed glob of tissue, the size of half a lime, was stuck to the muscle of her shoulder, under her skin. I looked around. Had anyone noticed? *A-ha* was still playing. I turned back to Emma. Her expression was the same.

But everything had changed. How had I not noticed the mass sooner? Now, under her wet, slick coat, it was obvious. My fingers instinctively palpated the area over and over, gauging the mass's size, texture, and adherence to other tissue. Maybe it's a lipoma, I tried telling myself—a benign fatty tumor that could be ignored—but I knew it wasn't. It felt malevolent, aggressive, cancerous.

At the clinic the next day I performed an aspiration, sinking a needle into the mass to obtain a sample of cells, a procedure I'd never imagined I would do on my own dog, regardless of its relative simplicity. I warily eyed the sample under the microscope before submitting the slides to the lab. The cells had large, violet-hued nuclei in a smattering of different sizes, and the cytoplasm swirled into a deeper blue pool seeming to flow from one nucleus to the next, making it difficult to distinguish individual cells. I didn't need a textbook; this was a sarcoma—a malignant soft-tissue tumor—locally aggressive but rarely to metastasize.

That same day we performed a CT scan of the area to gauge the extent of the mass. I didn't call Rob to get his permission, even though this had not been part of the plan we'd discussed that morning before I'd left with Emma. It was a quick procedure that could be performed under sedation, and it was what I needed to do. I hadn't forgotten the terrible night after she'd been sedated for her blood donation years earlier, but this was different. This was for her, to help her. Wasn't it?

The CT showed that the mass originated under her shoulder blade, and the hard half a lime I'd found was the tiny manifestation of a tumor that had burrowed its way from underneath her scapula to reveal itself when it was already too late. I was a specialist in hidden disease. I examined the function of internal organs sequestered deep in the body, diagnosed cancers invisible to the naked eye. This was what I did every day. This was what I had trained a lifetime to do.

There were three options, I explained to Rob later that night while Emma whined and paced the living room floor, groggy and anxious while the sedation from her CT scan wore off: limb amputation, palliative radiation, or do nothing. I looked at her graying face. *Was I brave enough to do nothing?*

We made the decision that night, quickly and decisively ruling out amputation—the only way to surgically control the cancer. I doubted she'd walk again if we pursued that route. Her right hind leg was too damaged to carry a third of her weight; it was already carrying significantly less than a quarter most of the time, judging by the wasting of her right thigh muscle.

I called the radiation oncologist at a local practice the next morning. "What would you do if she were your dog?" I asked, already knowing the answer. Radiation therapy, he replied without hesitation, a palliative course, five days of treatment, to slow tumor growth and improve prognosis. "This is what we should do," I told Rob later that day, talking to him like a client. "She can come home every day and she'll only need a short anesthesia." That she hated being in a cage, and being alone, that she'd always handled anesthesia poorly, were negatives I was willing to accept, and, I suggested, Rob should, too. He didn't question my decision; I was still the one to choose when it came to our animal family.

The following week we drove her an hour each way, for five days, to receive radiation therapy. She whined and barked when she was put into her run after treatment each day until she secured a spot under the lead technician's desk where she quietly napped. When we got her home she wouldn't eat, and we had to coax her with rice and cottage cheese, sweet potatoes, and canned tuna. The area of hair clipped over her shoulder was so much bigger than the small mass we could see—the hair took a long time to grow back, and when it did, it was the gray-white of her muzzle.

But then life pretty much returned to normal. And it stayed that way for a year or so. We didn't notice, at first, that we'd stopped walking everywhere with her. Or that her left front leg would tremble every time she squatted to urinate. Or even that the muscles of her right hind leg were melting away.

By the time her radiation therapy had faded to history, the tumor was growing again, wrapping its fingers of cancerous cells around her scapula, edging up toward her spine and forward along her neck. We had to make another decision. Should we try to repeat radiation therapy? Try again to slow tumor growth and buy extra time? But the outcome was now less certain, the probability of side effects higher. Radiation was not the right choice this time, we decided.

We started pain medications, adding more when the efficacy of the first waned. We limited her walks and our expectations. There had been a time when taking her on a walk annoyed me. Her attitude toward a neighborhood outing was always so lackadaisical; she wanted to spend too long sniffing the grass; she couldn't make up her mind where to pee. But then, when her collar chafed against the mass and she no longer pulled on her leash, when she would stop with her head down, panting, waiting for the pain or exhaustion to pass, I missed those walks with her that had once been so exasperating.

Those walks were normalcy. She had been Emma, not Sick Emma. I'd never thought of this when I instructed an owner not to walk their sick dog, whose heart or lungs were too fragile for exertion. I was strict: "No, not more than five minutes, no hills, no stairs. Only out to pee and straight back in." I hadn't understood what my prescription had taken away.

Her mass had reached the size of inclusion in polite conversation, and, as her owner, I was forced to explain her disease over and over. Hiding my sadness behind a smile, patiently explaining why we couldn't "just remove it." Purposefully not disclosing my profession to strangers, preferring to inhabit the persona of Emma's owner, not her veterinarian. I had never been so viscerally and tangibly confronted by a disease.

When the year turned into 2016, and Emma was still wagging her tail, eating well, and hopping onto the couch in the evening, it was easy to justify her still being a part of our family. But when she'd sometimes wake up stiff, reluctant to go downstairs, and less active—

moving only when she had to—I questioned if her life was as good as her tail-wagging made me believe.

But she keeps going, still hoovering up cat food off the floor when my back is turned, stubbornly and preposterously jumping into the car without help, still sleeping in the armchair she commandeered when she first came home. She has forced me to acknowledge that science is not enough. That the veterinarian I once wanted to be is far from the veterinarian I am. And that the only way to get there was to make the journey, no matter the challenges.

Every time I look at Emma I am confronted by a disease I cannot cure, a disease that is going to kill her. And the loss is not only in the futility of being a veterinarian who cannot save my own pet; it is in the knowledge that, although I can take what she has taught me and use it to treat my patients and build relationships with new animals in my family, I will never rekindle the particular love we shared once she is gone. This love, and the love each of us experiences for those we take care of, whether human or animal, is greater and deeper than anything science can teach.

# Acknowledgments

I'd like to thank my mum and dad, who have provided limitless support and encouragement for all of my and my sister's endeavors—ranging from hamster husbandry to trampolining to writing. Thank you for always believing that I could do anything I set my mind to. This story would not exist without you. And I would like to thank my sister for always "letting" me sit behind the driver.

Thanks also go to Tish McAllise Sjoberg, who reminded me how much I love writing and started me on this journey five years ago.

For taking a chance on a vet who wanted to write, thanks to Tod Goldberg, Agam Patel, Mark Haskell Smith, David Ulin, Emily Rapp Black, and the faculty and students of the MFA program in Creative Writing and Writing for the Performing Arts at the University of California, Riverside–Palm Desert.

I am indebted to my dear friend and writing partner, Kit-Bacon Gressitt, whose wisdom and generosity are limitless. And to Maggie Thach Morshed, the best cheerleader and friend a girl could ask for.

Annie and Ian McKie, thank you for introducing me to the magic of the Forest of Dean and for sharing your idyll.

My agent, Mary Evans, has guided this book from the very beginning, answered endless questions, and introduced me graciously to the literary world—thank you.

At Spiegel & Grau and the Penguin Random House Group, thank you to Julie Grau, Laura Van der Veer, Annie Chagnot, Janet Wygal, and everyone who helped usher this book into being. I couldn't have been in better hands.

It would be impossible to individually thank every student, intern, resident, technician, receptionist, teacher, and colleague who has impacted my life as a veterinarian, but I am grateful to you all.

To my clients, some of whom I've known for a day and some for a decade, thank you. And to my patients, who will never read this book, thank you for everything you have given me. Well, everything except the ringworm.

Cheers to the myriad people who have propped me up, pulled me together, and kept me going, even when I didn't deserve it.

Finally, I'd like to thank my husband, Rob, to whom I owe an endless debt of children's-birthday-party-and-swimming-lesson attendance, and without whom our family would have disintegrated from neglect while I wrote this book. There are no words to describe what you and our daughter have given me.

Thank you.

## ABOUT THE AUTHOR

SUZY FINCHAM-GRAY is a veterinarian and board-certified small-animal internal medicine specialist. She works in private practice, where she takes care of cats and dogs with complex medical problems. When pressed, she admits to being a cat person, but dogs come in at a close second. She holds an MFA in creative writing and writing for the performing arts from the University of California, Riverside–Palm Desert. She lives in San Diego with her husband and daughter, three cats, and two dogs. Her extended family still live in England, but they often visit with suitcases crammed with Marmite. *My Patients and Other Animals* is her first book.

## ABOUT THE TYPE

This book was set in Dante, a typeface designed by Giovanni Mardersteig (1892–1977). Conceived as a private type for the Officina Bodoni in Verona, Italy, Dante was originally cut only for hand composition by Charles Malin, the famous Parisian punch cutter, between 1946 and 1952. Its first use was in an edition of Boccaccio's *Trattatello in laude di Dante* that appeared in 1954. The Monotype Corporation's version of Dante followed in 1957. Though modeled on the Aldine type used for Pietro Cardinal Bembo's treatise *De Aetna* in 1495, Dante is a thoroughly modern interpretation of that venerable face.